instant
beauty

ALSO BY DEBORAH S. SARNOFF, M.D., AND JOAN SWIRSKY, R.N.

Beauty and the Beam:

Your Complete Guide to Cosmetic Laser Surgery

Deborah S. Sarnoff, M.D.

Robert H. Gotkin, M.D.

Joan Swirsky, R.N.

instant

*getting gorgeous
on your lunch break*

beauty

ST. MARTIN'S GRIFFIN
NEW YORK

www.stmartins.com

Design by Jennifer Ann Daddio

Illustrations by Elana Hayden, Hayden Web Design,
used with permission.
Web site: www.haydenwebdesign.com
E-mail: eh@haydenwebdesign.com

Library of Congress Cataloging-in-Publication Data

Sarnoff, Deborah S.
    Instant beauty : getting gorgeous on your lunch break /
Deborah S. Sarnoff, Robert H. Gotkin, and Joan Swirsky.
        p. cm.
    Includes index.
    ISBN 0-312-28697-X
    1. Surgery, Plastic. 2. Lasers in surgery. 3. Beauty,
Personal. I. Gotkin, Robert H. II. Swirsky, Joan. III. Title.

RD119 .S273 2002
617.9'5—dc21

                                            2001058904

First Edition: May 2002

10 9 8 7 6 5 4 3 2 1

To our wonderful son, William Ross,

our instant beauty from the day

he was born, whose favorite

school subject, in spite of

dazzling marks, is lunch!

D.S.S. and R.H.G.

To my "gorgeous" husband, Steve,

my "beautiful" children, Seth (and Jody Gerson),

David, and Karen, and my divine grandson,

Julian, who all appreciate that good

looks have their place but a good

character is forever.

J.S.

contents

part one:
the latest, greatest news!

part two:
a more fabulous-looking you!

part four:
instant beauty and beyond

illustrations

acknowledgments

We thank Sally Richardson, publisher of St. Martin's Press, for her enthusiastic embrace of our book.

We thank Michael Denneny, our editor, for his good nature, sage suggestions, and excellent editorial advice.

We thank Elana Hayden for her tireless research, heroic patience, and excellent graphics.

We thank Brigid Sweeney for her expert demonstrations of many of the techniques described in this book.

We thank the amazing Sara Hasty for her faster-than-the-speed-of-light medical transcribing skills.

We thank our patients, who put their trust in us and continue to make it all worthwhile.

And heartfelt gratitude goes to our families for their unending support and encouragement.

note to the reader

Medicine and science are now changing at the speed of light. Our intention in writing *Instant Beauty: Getting Gorgeous on Your Lunch Break* was to educate and entrust our readers with information and strategies to be used *with* but not *instead of* the decisions arrived at with their doctor. We trust that our book will inform readers about both the risks and benefits of "instant" cosmetic surgery and procedures and guide them to make informed decisions about whichever procedure(s) they choose.

Be aware that most studies are conducted by the manufacturers of skin-enhancement products and laser (or light-source) machines who have a vested interest in the outcomes. Negative outcomes are rarely reported. Short-term studies reporting on a brand new laser are followed by a lot of hype and hoopla in the media. Unfortunately, long-term studies are often still waiting to be done to prove a laser's effectiveness.

The vignettes we've used to illustrate different cosmetic procedures and treatments were based on composites of real-life patients. Any resemblance to any one individual is purely coincidental.

In describing fees for a particular procedure, we have given a range of costs that are generally based on geography, the reputation of the practitioner, and also the "hidden costs" of the facility and technology that are used. We have mentioned a number of brand name products and machines that provide cosmetic enhancements because they are used so commonly by doctors and aestheticians to describe this or that procedure, not because we endorse or have financial interests in any of them.

preface

In 1998, we wrote *Beauty and the Beam: Your Complete Guide to Cosmetic Laser Surgery* (www.beautyandthebeam.com), which spelled out the new world of laser machines and their ability to allow average people—not just the rich and famous—to utilize the latest technology to enhance their looks and correct cosmetic problems, among them aging skin, disfiguring port-wine stains, unsightly leg veins, unwanted tattoos, and the like.

The overwhelming responses were of relief and gratitude. This feedback didn't surprise us, although decades of feminist thought, psychological theory, and "values clarification" have insisted that what really counts in human interactions and character development is "inner beauty." Indeed, moral fiber and good deeds are infinitely more important than flawless skin, in fact paramount in moving society on an upward trajectory. But the wholesale discounting of outer beauty is more a function of lofty thinking than of reality.

In our new century, the retro debate about the relative value of substance over image has gone by the wayside. Everyone—from artists to athletes, doctors to decorators, politicians to professors, investors to Internet entrepreneurs, stay-up-late moguls to stay-at-home moms—recognizes that being honorable, productive, and successful *and* looking terrific are not mutually exclusive but rather perfectly complementary.

In our global and extremely competitive marketplace, where images on the Internet and TV as well as in the print media assail us daily, there is no question that appearance counts. While brains and energy remain at a high premium, the pressure for qualified people to look as young as they feel is more intense than ever.

People who are now living to hale and hearty old ages don't want to be held back because their looks don't correspond to their talents or motivation. In an age when physical fitness and good nutrition are part of practically everyone's life plan, people who feel vigorous and youthful but look tired and old want more equity between their inner selves and the packages they're wrapped in. And let's not overlook the good feeling that comes from simply looking good.

Gone are the days when people who didn't like their appearance spent years in psychotherapy delving into their self-esteem "issues" or lying about their attempts to look better. Today, people brag about their facelifts, nose jobs, liposuction, and laser peels. And why shouldn't they?

It's no fun to feel like a million dollars physically but look a decade or two older than your actual age, to be mistaken for your kid's grandparent, or to discover that the wolf whistle that turned your head was not for you. And it's downright demoralizing to get passed over for a job, be left out of a social scene, or look in the mirror each day hating this wrinkle, that blemish, or any number of cosmetic "defects."

No one has to hate his or her appearance anymore! While the cosmetic laser surgery we wrote about several years ago elaborated on the improvements in all aspects of getting gorgeous—from preparation to the bloodless procedures themselves to the reduced period of downtime—technology has advanced in such startling ways since then that just about everything we described has improved. Today, you can really get gorgeous faster than ever—even on your lunch break!

We hope that *Instant Beauty* guides you in asking all the right questions, critically evaluating the hype surrounding today's beauty products and services, and making wise and informed choices about the enhancement procedures you desire.

Deborah S. Sarnoff, M.D.
Robert H. Gotkin, M.D.
Joan Swirsky, R.N.

part one

the latest, greatest news!

instant beauty in an instant world

why getting gorgeous in a
nanosecond makes sense

"I believe in getting gorgeous," you may say, "but I simply don't have the time!" Even five years ago, this disclaimer had merit. While cosmetic enhancements were plentiful, they *did* take time, often involving weeks or even months of recovery. But that was then. Today, everything in our busy, fast-paced, multitasked, do-it-yesterday lives is done on the nanosecond clock—and the marketplace has responded.

Fast-food restaurants that once accelerated delivery with drive-through windows now promise a free lunch if the wait is longer than ninety seconds. And cooking, fuhgedaboudit! Instant meal services—either E-menus, eating out, or what takeout habitués call HMRs (home meal replacements)—are flourishing. According to a 2000 Zagat Restaurant Survey, residents of Houston lead the nation in eating out 4.9 times a week, with New Yorkers leaving their kitchens only 3.2 times a week, lagging behind the national average of 3.8 times weekly.

In addition, spas that once offered leisurely time-outs now

offer massages "on the run." Buses to the Hamptons on which passengers used to engage in catch-up conversations now offer manicures, pedicures, and hair-salon services. The Banana Republic offers to recharge your cell phone while you shop! And on-the-go, well-heeled and cared-for women, in a vanity version of the Tupperware or Avon party, now kill two birds with one stone by meeting at their dermatologists' offices for both social fun and quick-fix cosmetic procedures. At so-called Botox parties, groups of friends can enjoy appetizers and wine along with their injections.

These and dozens of other market-driven ventures are themselves driven by high-octane, 24/7 men and women who feverishly conduct stock transactions while they're sweating on a treadmill, speak on cell phones while they're driving, watch split-screen TV, send and receive multiple instant messages on high-speed computers, speed-dial and power-walk so as not to waste a second, have their feet massaged while their teeth are being drilled, and subscribe to dating services like It's Just Lunch or speed-date for a full ten minutes to decide if the stranger sitting across from them is worth more time.

In other words, people are in a rush to do it all and have it all—now!

The booming economy of the 1990s started this frenzy, and anxiety about the sluggish economy of the new millennium has no doubt kept it alive. The end of 2001 marked a period of economic slowdown in many retail markets, with the added impact of the disastrous World Trade Center tragedy. As one would expect, demand for more invasive and expensive procedures such as facelifts *decreased* dramatically because people were occupied with other concerns. Amazingly, the demand for quick-fix cosmetic procedures continued on an upward trend. According to one plastic surgeon, "After September 11, everyone felt out of control, and about the only thing people could control was the way they looked."

During the week of November 12, 2001, *CNN: Headline News* reported that spas across the country experienced increased bookings and expanded waiting lists. The Plastic Surgery Company, which owns and operates a national chain of cosmetic surgery and cosmetic laser centers, generated a 3 percent revenue increase in the third quarter of 2001 over the third quarter from 2000. They reported increased demand for physician-directed procedures such as Botox and collagen treatments. Since September 11, 2001, people may be canceling winter vacations because of security concerns and postponing purchasing large items such as a car. But people are still willing to splurge for a respite from the stress and trauma that has become a fixture in their lives. Psychologists tell us that during times of stress and uncertainty in the world, there are profound needs to find solace in activities that make us feel better and cared for. Many people feel that if they look better, they will feel better too.

In fact, it is interesting to learn that the sale of cosmetics doubled during World War II. When things were chaotic, there was some need for normalcy. When income was compromised, expenditures on less costly items or pleasures were substituted; even the danger of war did not dampen the desire to look good.

Nowadays, all of us, it seems, feel pressure to juggle the demands of our careers with the care of our children as well as time for ourselves and each other and also vacations. The net result is that everyone expects instant everything: instant happiness, instant potency, and also instant banishment of wrinkles. Hence the bonfire proliferation of "lifestyle" drugs like Prozac, Viagra, and Renova. But ahead of them all may be the desire for instant beauty!

Striving toward eternal youth—or at least an eternally youthful appearance—is no longer restricted to Hollywood stars or the very rich. Simple observation makes it clear that people of every age and economic status are now availing themselves of cosmetic quick fixes, from TV personalities to elected officials to the average Joe and Jane to those past eighty (the fastest-growing age group in the nation). Even the new "ruling class" of Young Turks between the ages of twenty-five and thirty are seeking a tweak here, a tuck there.

Leading the pack are the post–World War II baby boomers, who have been largely credited with spearheading society's keen interest in youth preservation and longevity through nutrition, exercise, stress-reduction techniques, and, yes, cosmetic enhancement. But they still worry about their appearances. A 2001 Roper-Starch worldwide survey about aging, beauty, and cosmetic surgery, conducted for the new AARP magazine, *My Generation*, revealed that many midlife baby boomers were suffering from self-doubt and feelings that their youth was fading. The majority of those surveyed said that when they hit forty-five, they stopped looking young. Mmmm. Perfect candidates for that "instant" cosmetic lunchtime fix!

In 2000, Americans spent $935 million for chemical peels, $235 million for collagen and Botox injections, and about $250 million for laser resurfacing. Nearly $1 billion was spent for facelifts and eyelid surgery. Of the billions expended, 250 percent more disposable income dollars were spent on cosmetic procedures than on movie tickets! That's not counting the nearly $1.5 billion spent on skin-care products.

This is not surprising. Since the beginning of time—in both the animal and human kingdoms—males and females have gone to great lengths to primp and preen in the evolutionary quest to attract suitable partners to perpetuate their species. Centuries before over-the-counter cosmetics existed, women painted their faces with the juices of colorful berries and indulged in aromatic baths laced with plant perfumes. And men pranced around in sexy loincloths and later waved scented handkerchiefs and donned elaborate wigs.

All this explains why both cosmetic surgery and enhancement techniques have flourished into multibillion-dollar—and growing—industries that are improving their products and services at such a rapid pace that whatever was hot even two or three years ago is just about passé today. Our supply-and-demand system and our pervasive race-against-time mentality have led us to expect—and yes, demand—cosmetic treatments that accommodate our increasingly fast-paced lives and are simpler, less invasive, and involve less downtime than even last year's products and services.

These expectations can now be met. In our brave new world of thirty-second attention spans, few people have the time or patience to experiment with avocado and cucumber lotions and potions, meditation techniques that promise "inner beauty," or lengthy surgeries that require protracted time off from work or play. In addition, many are simply not interested in going under the knife, considering it too radical, too risky, and too expensive. In truth, most people are not *that* dissatisfied with the way they look!

The good news is that medicine has caught up to their needs. Today instant beauty is available to everyone who has a lunch break to fix this, improve that, and get gorgeous! How is this possible?

- Big procedures have gotten smaller. Lasers that target problem areas with amazing precision and minimally invasive endoscopic surgery performed through tiny incisions both result in significantly less discomfort and scarring and quicker recovery.
- More than half of all cosmetic procedures—and *every* instant beauty procedure—are performed in a doctor's office or ambulatory surgery facility instead of the hospital, which offers patients more comfort, convenience, and privacy, as well as less risk of infection.

- Most lunchtime procedures require no anesthesia at all or only a topical anesthetic or injection for local numbing, allowing patients to undergo multiple procedures at one time and get right back to work or play.

For those who desire a quick fix—not just the "ladies who lunch" but also hungry men with hearty appetites—there is now an unending list of lunchtime procedures that can be performed literally in an hour or less and involve few if any side effects, reasonable cost, and immeasurable satisfaction.

Whether you are younger or older, these "instant" procedures will improve your outer self, enhance your confidence and self-esteem, and allow you to be competitive in your work and social lives. And every procedure we describe usually takes less time than your morning routine of showering, brushing your teeth, getting dressed, and starting your day.

While it is true that many lunchtime procedures can enhance your appearance and make you look better on the surface, these nonsurgical cosmetic tune-ups are not equivalent to a facelift that can correct sagging muscles and skin. However, a *series* of lunchtime procedures, each one leading to a subtle improvement, can cumulatively make a significant change in the texture of your skin and your overall appearance as well as delaying the need for a facelift.

Again, many of the procedures described in this book are not one-shot deals but rather packages of treatments that take place weekly, biweekly, or monthly. Because each procedure alone will result in only minimal changes, a series of treatments is often necessary to do the trick.

Just as most people have an interest in preventive strategies to keep them fit and well—and consider them well worth the price—many now recognize that cosmetic preventive strategies do the same, giving them the same psychological lift as do routine hair coloring, manicures, and pedicures. And just like these short-lived boosts to self-esteem, cosmetic enhancements work their magic for enough time to make you feel like the proverbial million bucks.

According to the American Society for Aesthetic Plastic Surgery, the top ten cosmetic procedures performed in the United States in 2000, in order of rank, were Botox injections, chemical peels, microdermabrasion, collagen injections, sclerotherapy (for leg veins), laser hair removal, liposuction, blepharoplasty (eyelid surgery), breast enlargement, and rhinoplasty (nose reshaping). All but rhinoplasty (which takes longer than a lunch break) are included in this book.

cosmetic surgery statistics

The American Society for Aesthetic Plastic Surgery (ASAPS) statistics on cosmetic surgery for the year 2000 estimate the total number of surgical and nonsurgical cosmetic procedures performed in the United States. The data were compiled by an independent research firm and based on responses to written surveys sent to nearly eight thousand physicians in three medical specialties: plastic surgery, dermatology, and otolaryngology.

procedure	number of procedures
Botox injection	1,096,611
Chemical peel	630,194
Microdermabrasion	610,705
Collagen injection	592,195

(continued)

procedure	number of procedures
Sclerotherapy	525,237
Laser hair removal	487,807
Lipoplasty (liposuction)	376,633
Blepharoplasty (cosmetic eyelid surgery)	212,133
Breast augmentation	203,310
Rhinoplasty (nose reshaping)	135,795
Laser skin resurfacing	116,901
Facelift	102,842
Breast reduction (women)	90,042
Laser treatment of leg veins	85,907
Fat injection	84,724
Forehead lift	60,756
Abdominoplasty (tummy tuck)	58,426
Cellulite treatment (mechanical roller massage)	51,253
Breast lift	45,710
Hair transplantation	38,978
Dermabrasion	29,905
Lip augmentation (other than injectable material)	21,266
Chin augmentation	20,499
Otoplasty (cosmetic ear surgery)	19,542
Male breast reduction	15,968
Thigh lift	10,357
Cheek implants	7,059
	(continued)

procedure	number of procedures
Upper arm lift	4,913
Lower body lift	3,362
Buttocks lift	2,122
Total	5,741,154

Statistics like these are objectively interesting, but to the person contemplating a cosmetic procedure, they say nothing of the consideration—and often anxiety—that goes into the decision to undergo a chemical peel or a Botox or collagen injection, among other cosmetic-enhancement procedures. Most patients (or, as they're called today, clients) have a million questions about what's hot, what's not; what works, what doesn't; what's fact, what's fiction; what's gimmicky, what's authentic; what's hype, what's the real thing. They want to know *what* each procedure entails and its cost, *who* is and is not a prime candidate, *when* he or she is ready for this or that procedure, *where* to seek the best practitioner and facility, and *how* to ask all the right questions.

In addition, they want—and have the right—to see before-and-after photographs that will help them visualize how the procedure in question may affect them.

To be sure, most people are already familiar with many of the cosmetic methods described in this book, having read about or seen them mentioned in any number of magazine articles and TV programs. But often what people read or see comes from the slick press releases of public relations firms hired either by doctors or by the companies that manufacture this or that machine or product.

Being mentioned is not enough! Any elective aesthetic procedure involves not only inherent risks but also the very delicate and ego-driven issue of personal appearance. No one takes this lightly and all people deserve to know *everything* possible about the choices they're making and the profound differences between the medical professionals and laypeople who offer the services they desire.

your skin, the sun, and your lifestyle

how to make people say,
"you glow, girl!"

We all know of great beauties with perfect skin whose inner selves betray shallowness at best or a lack of character at worst, just as we know of homely people with unattractive skin who distinguish themselves through good deeds or notable accomplishments. But the problem with stereotypes is that they're often riddled with contradictions. Beautiful people are just as often wise and beneficent as homely people are superficial or mean-spirited.

Whatever their traits, the common denominator of *all* people is that their skin is the first thing other people notice and, for better or worse, react to. Especially in our image-driven age, outer appearance is perhaps the most driving force of all, which is why literally millions upon millions of people are now availing themselves of skin-enhancement treatments and, for the most part, thanking their lucky stars that they did.

Before performing any cosmetic procedure, doctors assess a person's skin type, not to determine if it is normal, dry, oily, or a combination thereof, but to evaluate the skin's tendency to tan or burn when exposed to the sun in order to predict who is and is not a candidate for a variety of procedures. This evaluation is made according to the Fitzpatrick scale.

Fitzpatrick skin types

Type I: Fair skin, red or blond hair, blue or green eyes, freckles. Never tans but burns and peels severely. Example: Celtic.

Type II: Fair skin, blue eyes, blond or brown hair. Tans minimally, burns severely, and peels easily. Usually fair-skinned Caucasians.

Type III: Fair skin, brown hair, brown eyes. Tans moderately, burns moderately. Usually most common in Caucasians.

Type IV: Olive or light brown skin, dark brown hair, dark eyes. Tans easily, burns minimally. Usual in Hispanics and Asians.

Type V: Dark brown skin. Tans easily, rarely burns. Usual in Indians and Middle Easterners.

Type VI: Black or dark brown skin, brown eyes, black or dark brown hair. Tans darkly and burns only after severe overexposure. Usual in black-skinned people.

---

your skin

No matter what cosmetic treatment you choose, it will concern the skin, the largest organ in the human body. Constituting approximately 10 to 15 percent of body weight and an area of about 20 square feet, skin is composed of oils, lipids (fats), nutrients, living cells, and even dead cells.

Moreover, this versatile waterproof organ regulates body temperature against excessive heat or cold, retains moisture to form a protective barrier against outside stimuli, protects us from absorbing too much water, selectively permits medications on patches to enter the system, releases waste products and salt and water through the process of perspiration, and prevents the dehydration that might take place if too much sweat escapes. And don't forget the skin's role as our most powerful sensory organ—to temperature, pressure, vibration, pain, and pleasure.

Even when layers of makeup camouflage the skin, this multifaceted organ remains the most conspicuous and dominant of all body structures. For those who have a keen interest in improving the appearance of their skin by availing themselves of the treatments or techniques described in this book, it is helpful to know what this amazing organ is all about. Here's a primer.

EPIDERMIS
This uppermost layer of skin is comprised of about twenty overlapping layers that constantly undergo the process of birth, life, and death. No thicker than a thin piece of paper, the epidermis's

the skin

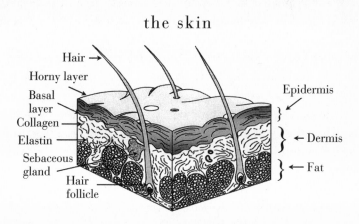

main function is to manufacture the protein keratin that enables the skin to act as a waterproof barrier and to protect us from superficial external injury. The epidermis also helps guard against harmful environmental influences like chemicals, pollutants, and excessive ultraviolet rays from the sun.

The top layer of the epidermis—the stratum corneum or horny layer—is made up of dead keratin cells that fall off when exposed to the environment or to friction created by washing or scrubbing. These cells are constantly replaced by actively dividing cells at the base of the epidermis, a process that takes about twenty-eight days in a person in her twenties but about six to eight weeks for someone in her sixties or seventies. When the stratum corneum is slow to replenish itself, the skin may appear dull and lackluster. Many lunchtime procedures, such as microdermabrasion or glycolic acid peels, target this upper layer to give the skin a radiant glow.

The epidermis also contains tiny openings called pores that serve as exit routes for sweat and oils and from which hairs emerge. While certain medications, chemicals, and toxins can penetrate the epidermis and be carried into the bloodstream, many other substances cannot. Contrary to advertising hype, moisturizers, collagen, elastin, vitamins, nutrients, and other agents that promise to purify, lubricate, nourish, tighten, or penetrate the skin simply don't reach its deepest layers, so their benefits are, at best, temporary and superficial. This is because no agent with a molecular size larger than water can penetrate the skin, and the molecules in most cosmetic compounds are too large to be absorbed.

The bottom layer of the epidermis contains basal cells (or basal keratinocytes) that are constantly reproducing. When damaged, primarily by the sun, the most common form of skin cancer, basal cell carcinoma, may develop. As they migrate upward, basal cells evolve into flatter squamous cells (also called keratinocytes) that make up most of the layers of the epidermis. Ordinarily, squamous cells migrate to the top layer of the epidermis, die, and flake off, but if they are damaged (again, primarily by the sun), squamous cell carcinoma may develop.

The epidermis is also the site of the skin's pigment cells, melanocytes, which contain the black pigment called melanin that accounts for variations in skin color. Melanin protects the skin against the sun's ultraviolet rays. However, chronic sun exposure can cause freckling and age spots as a result of an overproduction of melanin. If melanocytes undergo uncontrolled growth, the deadliest form of skin cancer, malignant melanoma, may develop.

DERMIS
This layer of skin is beneath the epidermis and made up of a tough matrix of collagen and elastin fibers that anchor and support the immune system's lymph vessels, blood vessels, sebaceous glands, sweat glands, hair follicles, and the pili erector muscles of the hair follicles that make our hairs stand up in goose bumps. The dermis also contains cells with nerve fibers that transmit sensations of touch to the brain.

The upper portion of the dermis, or papillary dermis, contains a vast amount of tiny blood vessels called capillaries that nourish the small arteries and veins and dissipate excess heat. After strenuous exercise, the skin flushes when the central nervous system sends an impulse to the blood vessels in the skin. In seconds, the vessels dilate to allow more blood to flow to the surface and be cooled by the outside air. It is from these blood vessels that conditions like rosacea, red-nose syndrome, port-wine stains, and hemangiomas derive.

The dermis also contains a dense network of connective tissue fibers, mostly collagen, which provide strength, and a smaller amount of elastin, which provides flexibility. Wrinkling and sagging occur when collagen is damaged and made more rigid by the sun, causing a similar effect as the creasing and bagging that tight jeans have when worn time and time again. The deepest wrinkles as well as ice-pick acne scars are found in the deeper level of the dermis, the reticular dermis. Stretch marks occur when elastin fibers elongate and break down.

SUBCUTANEOUS FAT

This layer, which lies beneath the epidermis and dermis, provides the body with energy, insulation, and an internal shock-absorbing capacity that protects against trauma. While "cellulite" is not a medical term, it is popularly understood to be the rippling, cottage-cheese-like appearance of subcutaneous fat that protrudes from the thighs and derrieres of women, to their everlasting dismay.

your skin as it ages

Even if you avoid the sun like the plague, your skin will eventually show signs of aging, not only from intrinsic factors like heredity and the inexorable march of time but also because of the lifelong workout it undergoes as you smile, laugh, squint, chew, purse your lips, and frown. All of these largely unconscious activities ultimately take their toll as collagen and elastin break down and the skin loses its strength and flexibility.

With aging, the skin thins, loses water, and becomes dry and less pliant. As it becomes more brittle and flaky, rough spots and scaly patches called keratoses may develop. The steady production of melanin that gives skin its color becomes irregular and may result in random whitened areas that look similar to confetti. If too much pigment clumps together, brown age spots appear, giving the skin a mottled or blotchy appearance. In addition, aging sweat glands cause a decreased tolerance for heat, and the diminished production of the natural oils in sebaceous glands causes increased dryness and roughness.

While the aging process may bring other changes as well—stiff joints, a slower gait, poorer eyesight, graying hair, forgetfulness, the list goes on—the skin remains one of the body's most resilient organs. Yet aging inevitably takes its toll on the skin, with the sun itself accounting for many of the blotches, mottling, wrinkles, pigment irregularities, dilated and broken blood vessels, leathery or parchment textures, and 90 percent of skin cancers.

your enemy, the sun

The statistics speak for themselves: more than a million people in the United States are diagnosed with skin cancer each year, nearly forty thousand with potentially fatal melanoma. Melanoma is now the most common cancer of women ages twenty-five to twenty-nine and second only to breast cancer in women ages thirty to thirty-four. Skin cancer strikes about the same number of people as all other cancers combined. Overwhelmingly, the culprits are the sun's deeply penetrating ultraviolet A rays that cause wrinkling, cataracts, and a lowered immune system, and the shorter ultraviolet B rays that penetrate the top layers of skin, damaging DNA and causing skin cancer.

Precisely why certain people get melanoma isn't known, but doctors concur that getting sunburned as a child or adolescent greatly increases your chances, as does being fair-skinned or having many (fifty or more) moles. Even one blistering sunburn as a child doubles the risk!

Yet in spite of decades of warnings about overexposure to the sun and the importance of sunscreens and sunblocks, beaches are overcrowded, convertible tops are down, and resorts are booming with sun-loving clients. Research studies about sunscreens are contradictory, some suggesting that they lower the risk of skin cancer, others that they confer a false sense of security that encourages people to stay in the sun too long, and still others that they do nothing to lower the risk of melanoma.

Nevertheless, American dermatologists as well as the American Cancer Society agree that Australia's "Slip, Slop, Slap, and Wrap" program is the best way to protect yourself: Slip on a shirt and other coverup clothing, slop on sunscreen, slap on a wide-brimmed hat, and wrap sunglasses around your eyes. Also think about avoiding the peak hours of 10 A.M. to 4 P.M. for outdoor activities, but if you can't, use an umbrella and seek the cover of shady trees.

Also crucial is applying a broad-spectrum sunscreen that blocks both UVA and UVB rays with a sun-protection factor (SPF) of at least 15. SPF, which is also found in cosmetics, creams, lipsticks, and lotions, is the increased allowable time of sun exposure before your particular skin type burns. Theoretically, if you're able to be out in the hot sun for thirty minutes before your skin burns, SPF 15 will protect it from burning for fifteen times longer—seven and a half hours.

It's important to apply an even coating of sunscreen, using about one ounce (about a shot glass full) for the entire body. People usually apply sunscreen unevenly, miss many areas of the body and, in fact, don't use enough sunscreen to protect themselves adequately. The result is that only 20 to 50 percent of the SPF listed on the bottle actually protects the skin. For instance, when an SPF 15 sunscreen is used improperly, the protection it confers can be less than 4.

Be sure to apply a sunscreen twenty minutes before you go outdoors to allow the product to bind to the skin's outer layer, and then reapply it every two hours since it dissipates with perspiration and exposure to water. A study conducted in Vail, Colorado, found that skiers who waited up to two and a half hours to reapply sunscreen were five times more likely to burn than those who applied it in two hours or less. Even if the weather is cloudy or cold or windy or snowy, 80 percent of UV rays reach your skin. Applying sunscreen to your face every day should be part of your daily self-care ritual. Why? Because the sun is always there! Even if you never burn again, a slight tan—the kind you get when you don't reapply sunscreen immediately following a swim—is still dangerous.

Wearing tight-knit clothing can also protect you from the sun's rays. An average T-shirt has an ultraviolet protection factor (UPF) of only 5, but manufacturers like Solumbra make clothing with a UPF of 30. Rit manufactures Sun Guard, a laundry additive that washes UV protection into clothes. The more you wash, the better it gets. After five washings, the UPF reaches 15; after ten, the UPF is 30.

One day sun damage and skin cancer risk may be eradicated by a lotion. A study involving thirty subjects, published in *Lancet* in 2001, described an experimental "morning after" skin cream, Dimericine, that repaired DNA damage caused by ultraviolet rays. But according to the researchers, no cream that is applied *after* the sun has already done its damage can substitute for adequately protecting yourself from the sun in the first place.

sun protection

There is no single "best" sunscreen or sunblock ingredient. Each product has advantages and disadvantages, which is why more than one sunscreen product is usually combined in commercial preparations to provide broad UV coverage and minimize unwanted side effects. Generally, people tolerate sunblock ingredients better than sunscreens, which may cause stinging, burning, or rashes.

Sunscreens are chemical agents that absorb the sun's rays. The ingredients that protect against UVB rays include:

PABA: May stain clothing and cause allergic reaction.
PABA esters (Padimate O and A): Rarely stain but may
    cause allergic reaction.

(continued)

Salicylates (homomentholsalicylate; octylsalicylate): Considered effective but may cause contact dermatitis.

Cinnamates (octyl methoxycinnamate and cinoxate): Insoluble in water and used in waterproof sunscreens. They are nonstaining but may cause allergies for those sensitive to cinnamon, tolu balsam, and coca leaves.

Sunscreen ingredients that protect against UVA rays:

Dibenzoylmethanes (avobenzone or Parsol 1789): Considered excellent protection, but some preparations may lose more than one-third of their potency after an hour of sun exposure.

Benzophenones (oxybenzone and dioxybenzone): Nonstaining but have poor water resistance.

Sunblocks are physical agents that scatter and deflect the sun's rays and protect against UVA and UVB rays. They include titanium dioxide, zinc oxide, talc, kaolin, bentonite, magnesium silicate, mica, or iron oxide. While perfect for the nose and outer ears, these opaque blocks can be messy and stain clothing. However, newer micronized sunblocks are virtually invisible and more cosmetically attractive.

your emotions

Just as noshing can temporarily satisfy your appetite, stopgap cosmetic measures can satisfy the outer image you entertain. But snacks don't compensate for a well-balanced diet any more than cosmetic quick fixes take the place of an actualized inner self. The importance of taking care of the inner self cannot be overstated, since even the most "successful" cosmetic lunchtime treatment cannot mask the tension, anxiety, or depression that arises from within and often diminishes—or negates—any superficial improvement.

If you're sad or mad or uptight, it shows! Even the most glowing skin, perfect hairdo, or dazzling outfit cannot eclipse negative emotions that reveal themselves in a clenched jaw, a dour expression, or the windows of the soul, our eyes. Or on the skin, which is the body's most "emotional" organ. Sweating, itching, hives, and exacerbation of skin problems like eczema, psoriasis, or acne often erupt during times of stress. Even when treated symptomatically, these unpleasant and often unsightly symptoms return when stress returns. Also rearing their heads in times of stress are bad habits.

When contemplating the plight of Darryl Strawberry, the New York Yankees star outfielder, or Ben Affleck, the Academy Award–winning actor and writer, or any of the other rich and famous people who regularly seek treatment at the Betty Ford Center and other rehab clinics, it is clear that drug and alcohol addiction are often more powerful and seductive than fame or multimillion-dollar salaries. Today, both scientists and society at large are inching toward the recognition that addiction— whether to cigarettes, drugs, drink, or gambling—is as much a function of biology as it is of psychology. New insights into the brain's chemistry as well as new drugs that target the brain's addictive centers hold promise.

In spite of addiction's intractable nature, it is also true that millions of people quit their habits each year through heroic self-control or by attending stop-smoking clinics or Alcoholics Anonymous, Narcotics Anonymous, Gamblers Anonymous, and Overeaters Anonymous meetings. Others—quite a few, in fact— are driven by vanity and manage to throw away their cigarettes the first (or second or third) time they read or hear that smoking makes them look older!

Cigarettes, of course, cause lung and other cancers and heart disease, and smoking doubles the odds of getting squamous cell skin cancer. The ingredients of cigarettes cause a breakdown of elastin and collagen, constriction of the skin's small blood vessels, and reduced blood flow that brings all nutrients to each cell of the body. The result is a lined "smoker's face," sallow complexion, vertical lipstick "bleed" lines around the mouth, and premature sagging, bagging, and wrinkles.

After years of heavy drinking, the blood vessels don't constrict, they dilate. Capillaries break down and cause a chronic flushing of the face. The reddish and purplish discoloration from the "broken" capillaries eventually forms a dense network on the nose, cheeks, neck, and chest.

To get the most out of any cosmetic enhancement, most health experts agree that it's important to replace stress and bad habits through a mind-body-spirit approach, embracing healthy living—an exercise regimen, a good diet, and peace of mind— by exploring the following strategies:

Short-term psychotherapy rarely revolutionizes your personality or character, but it often provides a change of perspective, new ideas about how to behave, help in sorting out your feelings, and emotional support that can catapult you out of a "stuck" situation. Psychiatrists, psychologists, nurse-psychotherapists, and social workers use various methods in short-term therapy, among them cognitive and behavioral therapy in which a patient learns to substitute new and healthier thought and behavior patterns for older, less productive ones, or an eclectic approach that includes elements of many different psychological schools. Remember that even the best-known or most highly recommended therapist may not be right for you. Trust your feelings and seek a new therapist if the first (or even second) one doesn't work out.

Note: Short-term therapy will not work if you're suffering from body dysmorphic disorder, a psychiatric condition seen commonly by dermatologists and plastic surgeons that is thought to be related to obsessive-compulsive disorder (OCD). In this case, the obsession is with the *appearance* of the body, specifically what's wrong with it, and the compulsion is to have more and more and more cosmetic procedures in order to fix the perceived defects. By and large, OCD is a glitch in brain chemistry that requires the appropriate psychotropic medications and supportive psychotherapy, both of which can help alter inaccurate perceptions as well as lessen the anxiety that drives this disorder.

Support groups are helpful for people struggling with a variety of conditions, both medical and psychological. Some are structured, usually led by professionals. Others are more free-wheeling, with members deciding on the topic(s) to be discussed. In all groups, confidentiality is an honored ethic.

Hypnotherapy is often helpful for people trying to break decades-old habits like smoking, as well as for overcoming phobias and reducing pain. Hypnotherapists, usually in forty-five-minute sessions, guide their clients into a state of deep rest that resembles a trance, although most describe it as a state of super-awareness. Some studies suggest that the limbic system, the structures in the brain concerned with the emotions, is stimulated under hypnosis to become open to suggestions that the conscious mind resists.

Biofeedback teaches people, again in forty-five-minute sessions, to become aware of normally involuntary body functions such as body temperature or blood pressure and how to control them through conscious effort. A machine measures skin temperature through a small sensor that is attached to the hand. By attaining a state of relaxation—stress cools the skin; relaxation warms it—and visualizing the blood flow that warms your body, you can bring about effective relief from chronic pain, elevated blood pressure, excessive sweating, irregular heartbeat, and migraine headaches, among other maladies.

Meditative techniques include transcendental meditation,

Zen, yoga, and other simple-to-learn meditations. You can practice them alone or in a group, and can even engage in them at home. Concentrative meditation involves focusing attention on a particular object or sound to quiet your mind and block out the external environment, while the goal of mindful meditation is to open your mind to sensations, thoughts, feelings, and images that may be overlooked in ordinary life. Meditation clarifies thinking and helps people enrich their spiritual lives.

Note: In all cases, learn the qualifications of the practitioner and if he or she is certified and/or licensed in this specialty. Meditation techniques are rarely covered by health insurance, but ask anyway.

A day at the spa, including a manicure, pedicure, facial, and full body massage, can provide the perfect antidote to a stressful week. The physical and psychological benefits of all this tending and polishing and buffing and rubbing cannot be overestimated. In fact, an astounding number of women who are juggling a million things manage to find both the time and money to indulge themselves routinely, and they always walk away with a clear mind, a clean body, and an uplifted spirit. But a spa or salon is the last place you should be treating yourself to a laser treatment or cosmetic surgery (see Chapter 4, "Better Safe Than Sorry").

Exercise is the only I-want-to-live-forever strategy that actually yields empirical proof of enhanced health. In addition to burning calories, exercise helps control blood sugar and cholesterol levels, strengthens the heart and other muscles, lifts the mood, clarifies thinking, and helps alleviate back pain, breathing problems, arthritis, poor circulation, and osteoporosis. And walking and swimming for people of any age is just about 100 percent injury free.

In terms of cosmetic appearance, exercise increases the blood flow that facilitates oxygen transport of nutrients that ultimately reach your skin and improve its color and texture. But the isometric facial "exercises" that promise fewer wrinkles do just the opposite! When you repeatedly tighten or contract your facial muscles, the skin develops more deeply etched wrinkles, much like the crow's feet that develop after a lifetime of squinting.

A balanced diet is generally described as a combination of protein, carbohydrates, a lot of fruit and veggies, and a little fat. Drinking plenty of water helps digestion, curbs the appetite, gets rid of body toxins, and keeps your skin well hydrated.

Interestingly, the Seven Countries Study conducted thirty years ago by Ancel Keys, Ph.D., of the University of Minnesota School of Public Health, revealed that villagers on the Greek island of Crete were found to have a 90 percent lower incidence of heart disease than Americans. Their diet consisted of whole-wheat bread, olive oil, beans, nuts, vegetables, fruits, and small amounts of cheese. They ate fish roughly once a week and meat (in two-ounce portions) about twice a month. They tended to exercise regularly and have strong family ties. Cancer was rare. Follow-up studies have endorsed this Mediterranean diet as a model for disease prevention. Americans largely agree with this formula but routinely violate it, perhaps because the embarrassment of riches we are offered in supermarkets and restaurants simply overtaxes our willpower.

In terms of the skin, research conducted at Baylor College of Medicine found that a low-fat diet (limited to 20 percent fat) significantly reduced the chances that premalignant skin tumors and subsequent skin cancers would develop on sun-exposed body areas.

Oral supplements like fat-soluble vitamins A and E may help to prevent or reverse ultraviolet ray sun damage, but too much vitamin A is potentially toxic to the liver. Vitamin C (important in wound healing), vitamin D, and the antioxidants selenium and beta-carotene are also protective. The hormones DHEA (dihydroepiandrosterone) that is produced in the adrenal cortex and melatonin that is found in the pineal gland are said to have antiaging qualities, but these (in fact, all supplements) should not be taken without consulting a physician or nutritionist.

The hormone estrogen markedly improves and may even reverse the skin's dryness, lack of luster, loss of tone, and deep wrinkling. However, hormone replacement therapy (HRT) containing the estrogen that alleviates menopausal symptoms is controversial because of its association with an increased risk of breast and uterine cancer. Only by evaluating her risk-benefit ratio can a woman and her doctor decide if estrogen is for her.

Whatever regimen you choose for yourself, keep in mind that the best antiaging strategies are a balanced diet that will keep your weight down, a regular exercise regimen, and giving up cigarettes and sunbathing forever!

CHAPTER THREE

what's hot, what's not, in skin care

fact, fiction, hype, and hope about the latest products

It's wonderful to have thirty or sixty minutes to "do" lunch or to combine a quick bite with a quick Botox shot, microdermabrasion treatment, Endermologie session, or superficial peel . . . the list goes on. Just about everyone has time for one or another or both. Except people who don't!

For those harried, hurried, don't-have-time people who are ravenously hungry as the clock strikes noon or one o'clock in the afternoon but simply can't take a break, hundreds if not thousands of take-out services provide the perfect alternative.

Fancy, the name she adopted because, she said, "Maryanne was so not me," was a quintessential New Yorker who never seemed to find the time to sit down to lunch. And like a lot of women who are born with great looks and great genes, Fancy could afford to be cavalier about her looks. The thirty-four-year-old blonde from Fairfield, Iowa, grew up on the campus of Maharishi University, the daughter of an artist mother and transcendentally meditating father who home-schooled her until she was sixteen "and fed me tofu and beansprouts." In 1989, a minute after she decided she had "learned enough," she took off for New York to make her way in the world.

"I always loved animals," Fancy said, "and had five big dogs, lots of cats, and littler creatures like gerbils and fish. I knew that my destiny was to care for animals, and when I hit New York there were a million people who wanted me to walk their cats and dogs, feed them, love them, take them to the vet, and even accompany them on planes to their second and third homes in Ibiza or Cannes or the Cayman Islands. I was so busy that I usually ate my lunch on the walk! All of a sudden, I started to realize that my pets looked better than I did, but I had no time to get as gorgeous as they were."

She confided in one of her employers, a woman her age who edited a glossy glamour magazine. "I could send you to one of the fancy cosmetics emporiums on Madison Avenue," the editor said, "but that would just be boilerplate advice. The best thing you could do is schedule a lunchtime 'vanity visit' with a dermatologist." She recommended a doctor and promptly made out a check. "My treat!" she said, adding that the visit would include not only advice about various products and an explanation of their ingredients but also a prescription for one of the FDA-approved topical medications if one was needed.

"Even more important," she added, "the doctor will give you a complete body check to make sure you don't have any suspicious moles that could be precancerous or cancerous."

Fancy immediately followed her advice and was surprised when the doctor told her that she had a mild case of adult acne and that some of the itching and flaking she had been experiencing was probably the result of the fragrances in the skin cream she had been using. It was only a matter of months after Fancy started using the medications the doctor had prescribed that she recaptured her once-perfect complexion.

"I was used to complete strangers stopping me to comment on how beautiful the animals were," she said, "so naturally I was thrilled when one or two of them actually looked at *me* and commented on my complexion!'"

In addition to having a dermatologist give you that all-important body check every year to make sure you don't have melanoma, it's a good idea for everyone to perform a self-body exam, as Fancy learned to do, every month and to follow healthy daily skin-maintenance routines.*

---

warning signs of skin cancer

Basal Cell Cancer

Symptoms: Pearly or pinkish patch or bump that is painless but may bleed.

Sites: Most commonly on the face, especially the nose, and the back.

Treatment: Freezing with liquid nitrogen, burning with electric needle, surgical removal when caught early. If caught later, more extensive tissue removal with possible need for plastic surgery repair.

Squamous Cell Cancer

Symptoms: May begin as precancerous lesion called a solar keratosis, a small, scaly red spot in areas frequently exposed to the sun.

Sites: Face, forearms, back of the hands. If not caught early may spread to other body parts.

Treatment: Freezing with liquid nitrogen, burning with electric needle, surgical removal.

(continued)

---

*Information about "How to Perform a Self-body Check," "Mapping Your Skin," and "The ABCD Warning Signs of Melanoma" can be obtained from the Skin Cancer Foundation at www.skincancer.org (see Resources).

Melanoma
Symptoms: Usually begins as a dark brown or black mole
    that may be variegated in color, with irregular margins,
    that may bleed when rubbed.
Sites: Any place on the body.
Treatment: Surgical removal. A total "body check" with an
    experienced dermatologist is the best hedge against this
    virulent, aggressive cancer.

daily must-do's

Just as you brush your teeth and comb your hair every day,
cleansers, moisturizers, and sunscreens should be included in
your self-care regimen.

CLEANSERS

Wash your face with a mild liquid cleanser rather than harsh
soap. Cleansers remove oily residue, makeup, dirt, and dead
skin cells without removing the skin's natural protective oils.
Never scrub your face. Wash it gently with lukewarm water once
or twice a day and pat it dry with a soft towel. Bathing dries the
skin more than showering, but whichever you choose, limit the
time you spend in the water and make sure it's not too hot. If you
have sensitive skin, avoid bath oils, gels, and bubble baths
because they contain dyes and fragrances. After your shower or
bath, apply a moisturizer to your entire body.

MOISTURIZERS

When applied right after a bath or shower to wet or damp skin—including the face, neck, hands, elbows, feet, and heels—moisturizers help to plump up and soften the skin and temporarily diminish the fine lines that inevitably result from bathing, exposure to the outdoors and the sun, certain medications, and aging itself. The main ingredients in moisturizing lotions and creams are animal fats (or emollients) like lanolin, mineral oils derived from petroleum jelly (such as Vaseline), vegetable oils, and vitamin E oil. Water-in-oil moisturizers, usually recommended for dry skin, are oilier and greasier and stay on the skin better. Oil-in-water emulsions, best for oily skin, are lighter and more pleasant to apply, but they rub off more easily.

If you can't tolerate oils, oil-free products containing silicone have a smooth feel. It's often difficult to tell from the label if a product contains silicone since the substance comes in many guises, such as cyclomethicone and dimethicone. Technical names aside, a silicone-based product is immediately recognizable by its uniquely smooth texture and fast disappearing act. Women with skin that is prone to blemishes find that silicone will not cause breakouts.

If your skin is sensitive, it's best to avoid moisturizers containing potentially irritating fragrances and preservatives. Manufacturers claim that the "natural" and "antiaging" ingredients in their products—for instance, collagen, elastin, placenta, aloe vera, olive oil, avocado, sea algae, and seaweed—will enrich, rejuvenate, revitalize, repair, nourish, firm, purify, or rebuild your skin. But collagen only attracts water to the skin; it cannot rejuvenate or replace the depleted collagen in your dermis because it does not penetrate. To truly replenish collagen, the protein must be injected and deposited directly into the dermis (see Chapter 6, "Getting Glamorous with Collagen Shots"). For the most part, the only thing a moisturizer does is lock in the moisture for a short period of time, so it needs to be applied more than once a day. Remember, it is not necessary to use moisturizers that cost $150 a jar. In truth, most products contain similar (or identical) ingredients, although their prices vary widely, depending on the hype of the manufacturer or the fancy packaging.

SUNSCREENS AND SUNBLOCKS

Both of these products protect your skin from the sun and help to prevent the sun damage that can lead to premature aging, wrinkles, or skin cancer. *Sunscreens* protect by absorbing the sun's harmful ultraviolet radiation. Sunscreens that absorb ultraviolet A (UVA) rays prevent damage to the immune system as well as photoaging (wrinkling and leathering). Those that absorb ultraviolet B (UVB) rays protect your skin from skin cancer and burning. Most broad-spectrum sunscreens that have a sun-protection factor (SPF) of 15 or higher are effective against both UVA and UVB radiation. *Sunblocks* like zinc oxide are thick, opaque creams that reflect the sun's rays away from the body. Both sunscreens and sunblocks should be applied daily, even on hazy days, and not only during the spring and summer. (See Chapter 2, "Your Skin, the Sun, and Your Lifestyle.")

Sunscreens and moisturizers are sometimes combined into a single product. For people on the run, this kind of product eliminates a step in the daily skin-care regimen. But if you apply a moisturizer with an SPF of only 8, it will do nothing to protect you at the beach. And who needs a sunscreen at night? Nevertheless, if you apply both sunscreen and moisturizer every day, there is a good likelihood that you will achieve similar and sometimes even superior reversal of sun damage as those who use antiaging medications like Renova every night.

pharmaceuticals

The FDA has approved the following medications after lengthy clinical trials. Some of them require a doctor's prescription. All of them have proved their ability to alter the skin's structure and function.

RETIN-A (TRETINOIN)

This is a topical medication derived from vitamin A that has been used successfully for decades to treat acne. When clinicians noticed that it also improved the appearance of fine lines and wrinkles, decreased the pigment-producing cells, repaired some of the tissue damage from the sun, and even reversed certain precancerous growths, they began using it for "off-label" cosmetic purposes.

RENOVA

This is really Retin-A in a moisturizing base and therefore helpful to people with drier skin. Although it will not eliminate wrinkles, repair rough or sun-damaged skin, restore elasticity, or reverse the aging process of the skin, it will smooth the skin, fade brown spots, and reduce fine lines and wrinkles, especially when used with a comprehensive skin-care routine that includes sunscreens, moisturizers, and protective clothing. *Before* any improvement is noted, there may be some redness, drying, flaking, and slight tingling of the skin, but these side effects ease over time. Renova must be used sparingly and, to prevent irritation, not applied on wet skin. Also, Renova may make your skin more susceptible to the effects of the sun, so it's important to apply a sunscreen with an SPF of 15 or greater daily.

If you are contemplating having certain lunchtime procedures, you may have to discontinue using Retin-A or Renova a few days prior because they may increase the fragility and sensitivity of your skin. These procedures include glycolic acid peels (see Chapter 8, "Feeling Refreshed with Chemical Peels"), microdermabrasion (see Chapter 9, "Rejuvenating Your Skin with a Power Peel"), or laser hair removal or waxing (see Chapter 13, "Laser Treatment of Unwanted Hair").

VANIQA

Vaniqa was approved by the FDA in 2000 specifically for the treatment of unwanted facial hair in women. The topical prescription cream contains the active ingredient eflornithine hydrochloride. Interestingly, it was originally administered intravenously to treat African sleeping sickness, and clinicians noticed that it also reduced the growth of facial hair. Vaniqa is believed to work by blocking a key enzyme necessary for hair growth and is effective for approximately 50 percent of women who use it. The cream is applied twice each day, but if the treatment is stopped, the benefits vanish! Women who use Vaniqa say that they are able to decrease the frequency of waxing or laser hair removal. (See Chapter 13, "Laser Treatment of Unwanted Hair.")

ROGAINE (MINOXIDIL)

This was the first FDA-approved medication to treat baldness or thinning hair. When it was originally used as an oral medication to treat high blood pressure, minoxidil was found to increase the growth of hair on men's foreheads, cheeks, and arms, leading to the topical formulation Rogaine. Rogaine helps men preserve their existing hair better than promoting growth. If it is not used indefinitely, the benefits cease. Statistically, one-third of men using Rogaine grow hair, another third grow peach fuzz, and the final third feel bad. Women have slightly better success with the drug.

PROPECIA (FINASTERIDE)

Propecia was FDA-approved in 1997 for the treatment of baldness in men. This oral medication promotes hair growth and preservation, especially when used along with Rogaine. There is a 2 to 4 percent incidence of impotence and loss of libido associated with the drug, but these side effects are much lower in younger men.

BLEACHING AGENTS

Hydroquinone and other "bleaches" slow or block the production of melanin to lighten age spots, fade blotchiness, and help erase dark circles under the eyes. When combined with Renova, Retin-A, or alpha hydroxy acids, hydroquinone is more effective. Over-the-counter fading creams like Porcelana contain 2 percent hydroquinone but are not particularly effective. Prescription bleaching agents with a higher percentage of hydroquinone (such as Melanex at 3 percent or Solaquin Forte and Eldoquin Forte at 4 percent) are more effective. Kojic acid (not a prescription drug) also lightens dark spots on the skin, as does azelaic acid (Azelex), a topical medication commonly used to treat acne. Overall, skin bleaches only lighten and fade dark spots; they don't remove them completely.

cosmeceuticals

Cosmeceuticals are a hybrid of cosmetics and pharmaceuticals. Unlike pharmaceuticals that alter the skin's structure and function and cosmetics that are intended only to beautify or enhance the appearance of the skin, cosmeceuticals may—or may not—have a clinical effect. While the FDA requires safety and effectiveness testing for drugs, no such requirements exist for cosmeceutical products. Except for testing the safety of color additives to gain FDA approval, and not including a few prohibited ingredients like hexachlorophene, chloroform, and methylene chloride, cosmeceuticals (and cosmetics) manufacturers are allowed to use any raw materials in their products. Cosmeceuticals like alpha hydroxy acids have druglike effects, but they are currently classified as cosmetics and thus are not regulated as drugs by the FDA.

The sales of antiaging skin-care products have made cosmeceuticals the fastest-growing segment of the cosmetics business, with an estimated $950 million spent yearly for antiwrinkle creams alone. While multinational corporations are ever on the lookout for new and improved plant extracts, minerals, proteins, and other promising cosmetic ingredients, their claims about their products' antiaging "miracle" properties are often exaggerated.

It behooves all buyers to remember that testing in laboratory flasks and on animals doesn't always translate to humans, and the long-term effects of this or that product are rarely known. Companies that manufacture cosmeceuticals sponsor their own studies, and therefore claims about their effectiveness must be taken with the proverbial grain of salt.

Despite the fact that the FDA requires labeling of a cosmetic's main ingredients, the beauty industry is loosely regulated and is not required to prove its claims. When you read that a product "improves the appearance of" wrinkles by 62 percent, for instance, it may sound very scientific, but it is far from promising to get rid of them. There is simply no way to know if a product that becomes the flavor of the month or a single ingredient that becomes the miracle du jour is more a function of company puffery than of genuine value.

Lately there seems to be a new fad every day for eliminating wrinkles, whether it be a new cream, a new oral supplement, or a new diet. There are even physicians who claim that after taking certain vitamins or following a special diet for only three or four days, you will see a noticeable difference in your skin. Misinformation like this is, indeed, misinformation.

CHEMICAL EXFOLIATORS

Alpha hydroxy acids (AHAs) are chemical exfoliators that derive from apples (malic acid), grapes (tartaric acid), sour milk (lactic acid), citrus fruits (citric acid), and sugarcane (glycolic acid). Low concentrations of these acids penetrate the outer layer of skin, peel away its horny cells, and deliver a uniform rosy glow, whereas higher concentrations penetrate the skin more deeply. An AHA with a lower pH (and therefore higher acidic content) is the most effective but often the most irritating. Buffered or neutralized AHAs are less irritating but still effective. Many AHAs cause a few seconds of mild burning and flakiness, which indicates that they are working. When combined with Retin-A or Renova, they are thought to accelerate skin renewal. They also help clear the skin of blackheads, whiteheads, and mild acne as well as lighten age spots. But claims that they stimulate collagen and improve the quality of elastin fibers have still not been proved. (For more intensive lunchtime treatments with AHAs, see Chapter 8, "Feeling Refreshed with Chemical Peels.")

Beta hydroxy acids (BHAs) contain salicylic acid, which has been known for more than a century to smooth the skin and eliminate scaling and roughness. It occurs naturally in willow bark, sweet birch bark, wintergreen leaves, and other plants. This and other BHA exfoliators are thought to have anti-inflammatory properties and are known to provide the same benefits as AHAs while being less irritating and causing less stinging and burning to the skin. They are a good choice for people with sensitive skin, mild acne, and/or a lot of blackheads. Stronger BHA solutions of 30 percent or higher increase collagen production and skin elasticity, but the higher solutions must be administered by a physician. Over-the-counter solutions of about 2 percent slough off the topmost layer of skin to give it a brighter appearance. (For more intensive lunchtime treatments with BHAs, see Chapter 8, "Feeling Refreshed with Chemical Peels.")

Polyhydroxy acids (PHAs), such as gluconolactone, are often combined with other hydroxy acids for the treatment of sensitive skin because they slow penetration into the skin of glycolic acid, thereby reducing stinging, burning, and reddening. In some products, PHAs are replacing AHAs because they have proved to be equally effective but not as irritating.

PHYSICAL EXFOLIATORS

Physical exfoliators are abrasive scrubs that target the rough, dry outer layer of skin, specifically the dead, horny layer of cells of the epidermis. Buf-Pufs, loofahs, oatmeal, ground-up nuts, apricot scrubs, and other granular agents—including, can you believe it, even diamonds!—are applied with washcloths to help exfoliate the skin mechanically. While all of these slough off debris, they can also leave the skin red, irritated, and in need of a moisturizer. (For more intensive lunchtime treatments using mechanical exfoliation, see Chapter 9, "Rejuvenating Your Skin with a Power Peel.")

ANTIOXIDANTS

Much of the oxygen we breathe is contaminated not only by normal metabolic processes but also by constant exposure to environmental pollutants like cigarette smoke and airborne chemicals. Food preservatives and, yes, the ultraviolet rays of the sun are also contaminants that affect our systems. The cumulative effects are cellular waste products known as free radicals, and they have been linked in numerous scientific studies to damage to DNA and RNA, autoimmune diseases, cancer, the breakdown of collagen in the skin, and other conditions or maladies. In addition, the normal aging process depletes the body of its own natural antioxidants, which may explain the higher incidence of illness as one grows older.

Antioxidants neutralize free radicals, and the best way to get them into your system is through your diet, especially foods that contain the most potent antioxidants: vitamins A, C, and E and beta-carotene. Antioxidants in skin-care products don't nourish the skin in the same way multiple vitamins do. To date, there is no hard proof that the antioxidants listed on moisturizers and vitamin creams (by their chemical names) live up to their claims of exfoliating the skin, stimulating collagen production, and preventing wrinkles.

In truth, the first-listed and most active ingredient in all moisturizers is ionized water! Research is now focusing on how to improve skin-care products so that the vitamins they contain can penetrate deeply into the skin. But don't forget that, ultimately, beautiful skin comes from a combination of a well-balanced diet and an overall healthy lifestyle that includes adequate sleep, exercise, plenty of water, no smoking, only moderate drinking, and certainly sun avoidance. Today, many of the antioxidants commonly associated with nutrition are found in all kinds of skin-care creams, sunscreens, cosmetics—the list goes on. They include:

Vitamin A is found in liver, fish, and eggs. Its derivatives, collectively known as retinoids, are the key ingredients in prescription topical skin-care products like Retin-A and Renova (tretinoin); Differin (adapalene), an acne medication; Tazorac (tazarotene), a psoriasis treatment; and the oral acne medication Accutane (isotretinoin). Retinoids help to repair and possibly prevent cell damage caused by free radicals, and also to minimize the signs of aging by lightening brown spots, smoothing rough spots, and diminishing fine lines and wrinkles. However, they may cause heightened sensitively to UV light and stinging and burning in people with sensitive skin. Doctors often recommend applying retinoid-containing products at night to avoid exposure to sunlight. Retinol, a form of vitamin A, is an ingredient found in many over-the-counter skin-care products. While it has a similar effect to the other retinoids, it's a less potent version.

Vitamin C, found in vegetables and citrus fruits, prevents damage by free radicals that could lead to skin cancers by offering protection against the sun and promoting anti-inflammatory effects. In topical skin-care products, the vitamin is found in the form of L-ascorbic acid and magnesium ascorbal phosphate. While claims of the vitamin's "magic" are persuasive, many clinicians believe the excitement about topical vitamin C is premature because of insufficient research about its ability to penetrate deeply enough into the skin to be of much help. It is still unknown if vitamin C can truly promote collagen synthesis and improve the skin's texture and firmness. In addition, some forms of topical vitamin C are so unstable in a jar that critics say they lose their potency the minute the jar is opened.

Vitamin E is found in nuts, seed oils, and dark green leafy vegetables. It is an oil-soluble antioxidant with anti-inflammatory properties that helps block cell membrane tissue damage. Vitamin E acetate is the form used most often in skin-care products. Before you run to open a vitamin E capsule and rub its contents on your scar, remember that like all topical vitamin preparations, those with vitamin E require more research before the medical community accepts them as legitimate healing agents.

Coenzyme Q10 is one of a group of substances known as ubiquinones that naturally occur in cells. Levels of the coenzyme decrease with age and can be further depleted by exposure to sunlight, ozone, and tobacco smoke, and also by psychological stress. This powerful antioxidant is found in numerous skin-care products ostensibly to scoop up free radicals and repair cumulative sun damage.

Other skin-enhancing antioxidants include green algae (flavonoids), lycopene (beta-carotene), ginseng, rosemary, juniper, gingko biloba, coarse chestnut, oatmeal, grape-seed extract, beta glucans (derived from oats and shiitake mushrooms), alpha lipoic acid, gluconolactone (the source of PHAs), green tea extract, and licorice root extract.

The jury is still out on the effect of antioxidants—including vitamins A, C, and E—when applied in topical potions. Yet there is considerable interest in the medical and manufacturing communities in combining these vitamins with sunscreens for protection against photoaging. When vitamins C and E are combined with oxybenzone, an ingredient that blocks out UVA rays, sun protection and antiaging appear to be enhanced.

VITAMINS THAT ARE NOT ANTIOXIDANTS

Vitamin B includes, among other nutrients, niacin, riboflavin, and biotin. While this vitamin is not an antioxidant, it is known to be essential in the normal functioning of the skin. Vitamin B_5 (panthenol) is used in some moisturizers and hair-care products as a humectant, attracting moisture to the skin or hair. One form of niacin, niacinamide, has been effective against acne when used in topical gel form.

Vitamin D is acquired from sunlight and absorbed into the body through the skin. Another source is milk and other dairy products. It is found in over-the-counter creams such as A and D ointment and in a prescription cream Dovonex (calcipotriene) that is used to treat psoriasis.

Vitamin K is often given orally to patients before facelifts and liposuction to improve blood clotting and minimize bruising. Though it is available in some cosmetic preparations, there is no conclusive evidence to date that it has these effects when applied topically. Nevertheless, it is widely marketed in creams that allegedly improve the appearance of spider veins and bruises.

TOPICAL HORMONE THERAPY

Wild yam extract (a plant source of progesterone), soy (a plant source of estrogen), and melatonin (a hormone from the pineal gland that triggers the sleep cycle) are antioxidant ingredients added to skin-care products to make the skin more supple. The tissue dryness that accompanies lower levels of estrogen is known to be correctible with estrogen patches or hormone replacement therapy, but in some postmenopausal women the risks of estrogen preclude its use. Several promising studies of the effects of topical estradiol (a form of estrogen) and of the less potent estriol on aging skin have been reported, but no double-blind controlled studies have been conducted. However, some studies have shown a small effect of hormone replacement therapy on collagen content and skin thickness in postmenopausal women. And one rigorous study reported that topical estriol reduced wrinkle depth and increased collagen production.

Another topical hormone, the antiandrogen Ethocyn, was introduced in skin-care products in 1995. Advertisements for this over-the-counter product feature split-face images of people with one side of the face wrinkled and the other side, the one treated with Ethocyn, dramatically wrinkle-free. Although the product is classified as a cosmetic, the manufacturer insists that it stimulates elastin production and results in smoother, suppler skin. Again, no large, multicenter, double-blind clinical studies are available to support this claim.

KINETIN

Kinetin (furfuryladenine) is an antiwithering agent found in the leaves of green plants. Early industry-sponsored studies at the University of California at Irvine and elsewhere indicate that within weeks to months of use, this cosmeceutical reduces blotchiness, fine wrinkles, roughness, and other signs of sun damage. Because it doesn't irritate the skin, many dermatologists prefer it to Retin-A, Renova, and other retinoids. It is sold under the trade names Kinerase and Kinetin and is starting to appear in many skin-care lines.

COPPER PEPTIDE

Copper peptide creams were first developed for burn victims and diabetics who had wounds that wouldn't heal. Today, cosmetic manufacturers are introducing copper peptides into various products to reduce pigmentation problems and wrinkling and to help the skin retain moisture. Early studies suggest that copper peptides produce more collagen than creams containing Retin-A, vitamin C, or melatonin. But be wary of studies released by a cosmetic company that manufactures a particular product.

cosmetics

Each year the cosmetics industry grosses several billion dollars in revenue from people seeking to highlight, color, camouflage, and moisturize their skin and enhance their features. Cosmetics contain hundreds of active and inactive ingredients, including emollients, emulsifiers, solvents, suspensions, humectants, thickeners, stabilizers, gellants, antioxidants, pigments, preservatives, and then some! Except for highly allergic people or those with unusually sensitive skin, most cosmetic products are so safe that the FDA does not require manufacturers to test them for effectiveness or list the fragrances they include.

For people who are sensitive, a variety of "hypoallergenic" products are sold that don't contain fragrances or other agents that might cause an allergic reaction. When you're reading the label of any product, "nonirritating" explains itself, "noncomedogenic" means the product will not cause blackheads, and "nonacnegenic" means that the product will not stimulate the formation of whiteheads and pimples. "Unscented" means the product has no odor, but it may contain a masking fragrance to cover the natural odor of the ingredients. "Fragrance free" means that perfume has not been added. Most products contain similar or identical ingredients, although their prices vary widely depending on the hype of the manufacturer or the elaborate packaging. The following products will do nothing but make you more gorgeous!

TONERS

Toners remove excess oils and temporarily "tighten" the skin. Also called clarifying lotions, refreshers, astringents, or purifiers, toners are appropriate only for people with oily skin or enlarged pores and should be used only once or twice a week. They don't actually shrink the pores, but their mildly irritating action causes a temporary swelling of the skin, making the pores appear smaller. Toners are not indicated for people with dry skin because their ingredients, like alcohol, witch hazel, salicylic acid, and resorcinol, can further dry the skin.

BRONZERS AND SELF-TANNERS

A bronzer is a self-applied cosmetic that gives you a sun-kissed appearance. It lasts about a day and can be washed off with soap and water. A self-tanner is a water-soluble cream containing a nontoxic dye (DHA or dihydroxyacetone) that binds to the skin's outer layer to produce an authentically suntanned look lasting several days. As the dead cells in the skin's outer layer slough off, the tan gradually disappears unless the cream is reapplied. While both bronzers and self-tanners may contain sunscreens with a low SPF, neither offers significant protection against the sun's rays, so it is best to apply a tanner at night before bed and use a sunscreen in the morning. For a more uniform look from a self-tanner, it is helpful to use an exfoliating agent beforehand.

Don't be misled by products that sound like self-tanning lotions, such as tanning amplifiers, tan accelerators, or, worst of all, tanning pills. These products interact with the sun to create a tan that actually accentuates skin damage. The pills, which are banned in the United States, have been associated with hepatitis and hives. Read the ingredients carefully. Unless the active ingredient is DHA, the tanning agent may be harmful to your skin.

MASKS

Masks have a base of clay or mud and are effective in removing sebum from oily skin and helping to unclog pores. Moisturizing masks with a base of cream or oil hydrate dry skin. When applied once a week, masks leave the skin looking smooth and refreshed.

FOUNDATIONS

Pan-Cake makeup is not used much anymore, but powders are still popular to cover facial skin. More common are the flesh-toned liquid agents that give the skin a sheer, smooth look. Whether they give the skin a matte (flat) finish or a pearlized shimmer, foundations are essentially moisturizers to which iron-oxide pigments have been added, and many contain a sunblock or sunscreen.

CAMOUFLAGE MAKEUP

Also called masking foundations, these flesh-toned products are thicker and more opaque than regular foundation and are used to camouflage scars, bruises, and discolorations. Usually oil-based, water-resistant, and long-lasting, they provide added protection against the sun.

CONCEALERS

Also called primers or neutralizers, concealers are not as heavy as masking foundations but are often used under foundation to counteract blemishes and neutralize pigment irregularities. They work like lasers, on the laws of the color wheel. For instance, complementary colors, when combined, result in the neutral color beige or brown; a yellow concealer will disguise purple skin discolorations, bluish bruises, and dark circles under the eyes; green will cover up broken blood vessels in a ruddy complexion and the redness that is evident during the healing phase following laser resurfacing; and purple will neutralize yellow bruises and sallow complexions.

The art of making up (as in enhancing your face) is both fun and satisfying, but it can't make your skin younger. In fact, when makeup becomes caked, deep wrinkles are exaggerated. The best hedge against premature aging is, as we've said, a healthy lifestyle and, of course, the lucky roll of the dice known as good genes.

With so many products on the market—some of them of dubious value but hyped to the hilt and others with more science to back them up but equally hyped—it is almost impossible for the average woman to know which skin-care product or cosmetic treatment is best for her. By and large, dermatologists who are trained and educated in all matters of skin disease and health are best equipped to read the science, evaluate its worth, diagnose, treat, and recommend.

Nowadays, your dermatologist may not only recommend a particular product but may also offer to sell it to you. Some patients are grateful for this one-stop-shop and consider the doctor more knowledgeable about skin than the lady in white behind the cosmetics counter at the department store. Others may feel obligated and even uncomfortable about what they perceive to be a conflict of interest. Remember, *you are under no obligation* to buy any product, no matter who recommends it. Patients themselves are the best equipped to determine what they want to do about their skin, if anything.

Whether or not you choose to buy products from your doctor, it is still a good idea to bring all the products you're currently using to your vanity visit in order to discuss them with your dermatologist and learn about the best skin-care and sun-protection regimen for you. Another good decision is to have a yearly "body check"—as you do a Pap test and a mammogram—to make sure that your outer self is in as good shape as your inner self. Both, of course, can be done on your lunch break!

better safe than sorry

*finding the safest facility and
asking the right questions*

Every day, newspaper headlines warn the public about this or that incipient threat to their health and TV anchors start the news with similar warnings: "Is what you are eating safe?" "Can salad make you sick?" "Don't touch that chicken!" "Is fast food deadly?" "Careful about that sushi!"

While alarmist in tone, many of these warnings are rooted in the frightening facts of modern existence: widespread outbreaks of salmonella and ptomaine poisoning, hepatitis, shigellosis and other, sometimes fatal, food-borne illnesses that come about from spoilage or unsanitary handling. Often, prevention involves just a few easy precautions like washing your hands after handling raw chicken, not eating raw meat, being alert to expiration dates, and the like.

It's not so easy, however, to ensure that the cosmetic procedure you desire will be performed at the safest facility or by the most experienced practitioner. As everyone knows, the medical world is also plagued by frightening facts, among them that medical errors account for thousands of grave injuries and deaths in U.S. hospitals every year in spite of the fact that the pledge *primum non nocere*—first, do no harm—is the most cherished ethic of medical practice.

For modern patients faced with these bleak statistics, better safe than sorry should be the driving criterion of all trips to the doctor, even if they're for elective procedures that are noninvasive and therefore considered "safe" and that are generally performed in outpatient settings. In actuality, any cosmetic procedure, no matter how quickly it's performed or how little preparation it requires, has inherent risks.

Putting aside for a moment the "instant beauty" subjects discussed in this book, consider the intractable fungus infections that many women suffer from having manicures and pedicures, most if not all of which might have been avoided by insisting on the sterilization of cuticle cutters, buying one's own instruments, checking that the operator is state licensed, or looking over the nail salon for simple cleanliness. How much more urgent, then, to check the credentials and facility of the practitioner who will be working on your face and body!

is there a doctor in the house?

Once upon a time, medical doctors were considered the only people capable of evaluating patients for various medical procedures, determining if any underlying problems existed, administering injections and medications, and providing follow-up care. Over the past decade or two, however, medicine has changed radically, as managed care and health maintenance organizations have forced hospital chains to consolidate, cut costs, and set tough restrictions on the ability of doctors to order tests and perform elective surgery, among other practices.

As doctors have been forced to beg untrained insurance clerks for permission to practice their own brands of medicine, many of them have begun to look for alternative sources of income—and satisfaction—by broadening their practices, becoming experts in "lifestyle" issues like diet, nutrition, and exercise, and marketing their own brands of vitamins and other supplements. Many have converted their traditional medical practices into more lucrative "wellness" centers or cosmetic practices where patients, who are now called "clients" or "customers," pay up-front.

The trend to branch out from their areas of specialty is so popular among physicians that vanity procedures like laser hair removal, microdermabrasion, or Endermologie are even offered by gastroenterologists, ophthalmologists, and obstetricians! Some doctors have opened satellite offices they never even visit themselves, relying on auxiliary personnel—and not always medical personnel—to conduct business.

heed the hype!

All this has resulted in doctors getting caught up in the big business of cosmetic surgery, with companies that manufacture skin-care products and laser machines plying physicians with packages of sophisticated marketing material, pitch letters, press releases, fact sheets, and glossy before-and-after photographs to help sell the cosmetic concept to potential patients. The result is that the high regard the medical establishment once enjoyed has been compromised. Today, there is a growing consumer movement of patients who are less interested in the old-time one-to-one relationship with their doctors than in comparison shopping for the best deal.

Caveat #1: When you read about cosmetic-enhancement treatments in popular magazines and they mention this or that doctor as "the best," be aware that this publicity may be the result of the public relations firm the doctor has hired and not a measure of his or her knowledge or experience with cosmetic procedures.

spa—skin protection alert!

It isn't only doctors who are climbing on the high-technology bandwagon of cosmetic enhancement. Competing with the very physicians who buy their machines, manufacturers of lasers and other equipment are now opening cosmetic spas and salons that feature their products, often hiring doctors as medical directors but not guaranteeing that they will be on-site during the procedures themselves. It's no longer medicine, it's big business and big bucks. In fact, some spas advertise that the first treatment is free. But as we all know, there's no such thing as a free lunch!

The price patients pay in terms of safety may be high. Spa or salon employees are neither educated nor trained to diagnose medical conditions. While the most highly trained aesthetician may complete six hundred hours of course work, preparation for most is significantly less. This is in stark contrast to the training of physicians: four years of medical school, three to eight years of residency in a specialty area, and often follow-up fellowships.

Simply, an aesthetician cannot be expected to determine whether excess hair results from a hormonal dysfunction of the ovaries or adrenal glands, whether prominent broken blood vessels on the face result from a serious systemic disease like lupus, or whether a cosmetically bothersome brown spot is, in fact, a potentially fatal malignant melanoma.

In addition, spa and salon employees are ill equipped to respond to emergencies like life-threatening allergic reactions or to distinguish heart attacks from transitory anxiety attacks. They cannot—and should not be expected to—distinguish between complications like herpes or folliculitis, which require different therapies. In many lunchtime cosmetic procedures, the potential for scarring, infection, and pigment changes cannot be underestimated.

Caveat #2: If you choose a cosmetic treatment in a spa or salon, insist that a medical doctor who is qualified in the treatment of the skin is present and supervising the procedure.

To check on a physician's board certification, training, licensing, specialty, or any disciplinary action, you can consult *The Marquis Who's Who Directory of Medical Specialists,* a series of volumes found in most libraries, or your state board of medicine. In addition, several on-line sites allow you to check the background, credentials, and "track record" of your doctor. They include the American Board of Medical Specialties at http://www.abms.org, http://www.trustmydoctor.com, http://www.docboard.org, and http://www.maxpages.com/doctorsreports. If you are seeking skin-care treatments in a spa or salon, be sure to ask the following questions:

- Who will be administering the treatment?
- What training in the procedure has that person had?
- Will a doctor examine me beforehand?
- Will a doctor be supervising the treatment?
- What is the policy of the spa if any complications arise?

questions to ask your doctor—and yourself

While the American Society for Laser Medicine and Surgery, the American Academy of Dermatology, and the American Society for Dermatologic Surgery, among other medical organizations, have published broad recommendations for laser practice, there are still no national criteria for laser training, no mandatory requirements, and no board examinations requiring doctors to become certified in laser procedures or surgery. A doctor who is familiar with one type of laser may be totally ignorant in the use of others, which could make the difference between a satisfactory or disastrous outcome. Be sure to ask your doctor the following questions:

- Are you board certified? In what specialty?
- What training and experience have you had in performing laser surgery on people (and not tomatoes or eggplants!)?
- What experience have you had in performing the particular procedure(s) I am interested in?
- Can I speak directly with other patients of yours who have undergone the same procedure I desire?
- Will you be available to answer my questions or concerns over the phone?
- Are the before-and-after photographs examples of your work, or did they come in the media kit supplied by the laser company?
- Does your facility have emergency equipment on the premises, and is your staff trained and certified in emergency procedures such as advanced cardiac life support, cardiopulmonary resuscitation, seizure treatment, and the like?
- What will the treatment cost? Is there a financing plan? Can I pay with a credit card? (In addition to the doctor's fee, there may be other charges for the laser, facility, or anesthesia.)

Even if you get satisfactory answers to all the above questions, you still need to ask yourself:

- Do I feel comfortable with and trust my doctor?
- Is the facility spotlessly clean?

- How receptive is the doctor to my questions?
- Is the staff receptive and friendly?
- Am I being honest with my doctor about everything in my medical history, including all the medications I'm taking (even aspirin!), allergies, the fact that I smoke, if I have a history of herpes, as well as problems with substance abuse?

Caveat #3: Failure to learn as much as possible about the procedure you desire and to be your own best advocate is not only foolhardy but also potentially dangerous.

is laser treatment safe?

Many doctors' offices and freestanding centers are not affiliated with any hospital and so are not regulated by state or federal governments and are subject only to random inspections by the Occupational Safety and Health Administration (OSHA). Except for a handful of states, including California and Florida, accreditation of such facilities is voluntary through the Accreditation Association for Ambulatory Health Care, the American Association for Accreditation of Ambulatory Surgery Facilities, or the Joint Commission on Accreditation of Healthcare Organizations (see Resources).

Today, doctors in most states can open an outpatient surgical or treatment center simply by meeting their state's safety code for similar facilities and developing written policies outlining procedures that will be followed in various situations. Considering the inherent risks of laser surgery, this "honor system" is not good enough.

The American National Standards Institute (ANSI), a consortium of manufacturers, trade associations, professional organizations, consumers, government and military agencies, and research and educational facilities responsible for establishing thousands of nonregulatory standards, has published a document titled, "National Standards for the Safe Use of Lasers in Healthcare Facilities." This guideline has become the national benchmark for laser safety. The key to safe laser practice, whether in a hospital operating room or a private medical practice, is application of the ANSI standards, which include the following:

- Eye protection. The FDA requires that each individual laser come with nonflammable, wavelength-specific protective eyewear (often goggles or wraparound glasses with side shields) for doctors, patients, and ancillary personnel. Even a small amount of reflected laser energy can harm the eyes or even result in blindness.
- Fire protection. Because a fire or explosion may result from either direct or scattered radiation, dry cloth or paper drapes are avoided and all surfaces including wall coverings are covered with fire-retardant material. A fire extinguisher should be nearby during all laser procedures and the surface of any metallic surgical instruments should be dulled. Reflective surfaces like mirrors and jewelry should be eliminated.
- Protection from transmission of diseases. Dangerous matter has been a concern of doctors and patients since portions of viral DNA from the wart virus, hepatitis virus, and HIV (the virus that causes AIDS) were found to be airborne in operating rooms, including in the CO_2 laser's plume and in electrosurgical smoke. Therefore, when appropriate, masks are worn, smoke is evacuated safely, and the laser room is protected from unauthorized personnel.

Caveat #4: For your own safety and peace of mind, definitely inquire if the laser facility you are considering is accredited by one of the above-mentioned organizations and if every safeguard is being taken. The laws on who can operate a laser vary from state to state. Fifteen states do not allow anyone other than a physician to perform the service, and many require a physician's direct supervision.

Overwhelmingly, people undergoing cosmetic enhancement with lasers, light sources, chemical peels, and other methods are thrilled with the outcome. But any treatment that involves either lasers or chemicals holds the same potential risks and requires the same kind of caution as driving a car, operating a microwave oven, or even cooking out on a gas grill.

Final caveat: Remember, you only have one face and one body! That is why, in choosing any cosmetic procedure, it is imperative to do your homework and ask a lot of questions, both of which will help you choose the right practitioner and the best facility.

CHAPTER FIVE

quick fixes

*all about ear piercing, permanent
makeup, and treating torn
earlobes, scars, moles,
and zits*

The old standard "Little Things Mean a Lot" referred to the small, endearing romantic gestures that make all the difference in a good relationship. But people who suffer from many "little" skin problems and cosmetic imperfections might interpret those words in a different way. Yes, they would say, these little things mean a lot to me every day—a lot of grief, a lot of embarrassment, a lot of aggravation.

Those little things no longer have to be tolerated. By selectively choosing among the quick cosmetic fixes that are now available, you can improve your appearance in little more than a blink of the eye.

Daisy, a twenty-five-year-old professional basketball player, was tall, slim, and stunning, with unblemished skin that still glowed and glistened with the blush of youth. Admired and envied for her career success and striking looks, she seemed like the last person to haunt a dermatologist's office. Yet she was in the habit of fixing lots of little skin problems, always to her satisfaction.

"Nothing I've had done was urgent," she said, "but I always figured, why wait?" Indeed, no one has to wait to get a little more gorgeous by correcting any number of minor but bothersome skin glitches. Here is a sample of some of the hottest procedures that can be performed on your lunch break.

ear piercing

New York and several other states have laws mandating that anyone under the age of eighteen must have parental permission to pierce any part of the body, but this is hardly the norm. Millions of ears, belly buttons, tongues, eyebrows, and other body parts are pierced every day in unregulated tattoo parlors, malls, kitchens, and who knows where else. What you don't hear about is the nasty infections that often follow these innocently undertaken procedures and the protracted suffering they cause. For maximum safety and to cut down your risks, it's infinitely wiser to have your ears (and anything else) pierced in the office of a dermatologist or plastic surgeon where OSHA standards and sterility prevail. (See Chapter 4, "Better Safe Than Sorry.")

Piercing takes only five or fewer minutes. First, your ears (or other body area) are cleansed with alcohol, the sites marked to assure symmetry, and a local anesthetic (or ice) administered to chill the area. Then the ear is pierced with a tiny needle or a pressurized gun, and topical antibiotic ointment is applied. Often, people want additional holes placed in their ears, which is fine. But be warned: There is a higher risk of infection for a hole made in the ear's cartilage rather than in the soft tissue of the lobe.

repairing a torn earlobe

After years of wearing heavy hanging earrings or dangling hoops, the pierced holes in your earlobes may become elongated or, in some cases, torn. And it's not uncommon for earrings to tear the earlobe when they get caught in a sweater when it's taken off over the head. Repairing the tear is a popular lunchtime procedure in which the earlobe is numbed with a local anesthetic and a scalpel is used to contour the damaged area. Sutures are placed in the skin and removed in several days. In some cases, you can wear a pierced earring immediately; in other cases, it takes more time, even months.

applying permanent makeup (micropigmentation)

Micropigmentation—or medical tattooing that utilizes the same techniques, equipment, and pigments as nonmedical tattoo artists—is the art of implanting small amounts of colored pigments into the skin for cosmetic adornment and camouflaging or reconstructive purposes. Pigments are combined and blended to match the color of whichever body part is being reconstructed or enhanced. Because there is no certification for the application of permanent makeup—which can be applied by physicians, medical paraprofessionals, aestheticians, and makeup artists—it's especially important to find a practitioner whose work you have seen and respect. The technique is utilized for a variety of reasons, including:

- For endowing permanent color on the lips, eyebrows, eyelids, and cheeks.
- For restoring color to white scars from burns, accidents, or prior surgery.

- For women with arthritis who are unable to apply makeup.
- For those with multiple sclerosis or Parkinson's disease, which affects the muscular and nervous systems and may produce tremors or unsteadiness in the hands.
- For coloring the nipple and the area around the nipple (the areola) on women who have had breast reconstruction after a mastectomy.
- For those with visual impairment or blindness who cannot put on makeup.
- For those with contact lenses, seasonal allergies, or sensitivity to regular makeup.
- For those with port-wine stains or other skin discolorations, flesh-toned tattoos help to mask their blemishes.
- For those with vitiligo, an autoimmune disease in which the body attacks the pigment cells and leaves the skin mottled with stark white spots, permanent makeup camouflages the spots to match the normal skin.
- For those who swim every day or live the "instant everything" life and don't have the patience to keep reapplying makeup.

Despite the advantages of micropigmentation, there are people who want their cosmetic tattoos removed. For the most part, removing cosmetic tattoos is like removing decorative tattoos (see Chapter 11, "Laser Treatment of Brown Blemishes"). But removing tattoos with a laser can be risky. Flesh-tone colors like tan, beige, light pink, light brown, rust, and white may instantly blacken because the iron compound ferric oxide in flesh-toned tattoos is changed to ferrous oxide, which causes the tattoo, paradoxically, to turn black. Consequently, the black tattoo becomes more difficult to remove and may actually look worse than the original. After multiple laser treatments, the blackness may dissipate but in some cases it is permanent. Complete excision or vaporization of the skin with a resurfacing laser may be the only remaining option in getting rid of the black pigment.

In most micropigmentation procedures, the area to be treated is anesthetized with EMLA cream or local lidocaine injections, after which the pigment is injected into the skin with tiny needles. Since the color is permanent, too little pigment is better than too much. In most cases, extensive pigment placement should be performed in stages over a period of weeks to months to allow the patient to evaluate each phase. Side effects include pigment migration, most common in eyelid procedures, in which tiny granules move along the ducts of sebaceous glands creating a "halo" around the eyelashes. Infection and scarring can occur if the micropigmentation practitioner is careless. Therefore, it is imperative to have this enhancing but potentially risky procedure done by an experienced practitioner whose office complies with OSHA standards and whose needles are sterilized to prevent the spread of both bacterial and viral disease.

You can have permanent makeup applied to your lips or as eyeliner on your lunch break, but the areas will become swollen after the procedure so it's best to call it a day instead of returning to work.

treating a big zit

If you have ever woken up to find a big, tender, red zit on your face, you know the horror! The whole world, you think, will not hear a word you say or appreciate the outfit you're wearing or value your wonderful qualities—they will only be looking at your gigantic pimple! Warm compresses may help, but they will not vanquish the nightmare in plain view. And topical antiacne medication, including topical antibiotics, won't work either because the pimple is deeper down in the skin. The worst part is that these kinds of zits won't go away on their own for two or three weeks. Well, here's the solution: Call your dermatologist and tell the receptionist that you're having a vanity emergency! The doctor will inject a small amount of the steroid Kenalog directly into the pimple with a tiny needle, and poof! Within twenty-four (or maybe forty-eight) hours, the pimple flattens and the inflammation diminishes significantly. The whole thing takes only a couple of tolerably uncomfortable seconds. One possible side effect is that Kenalog may cause a *temporary* indentation at the site of the injection if the dosage is too strong, but most doctors dilute the steroid with saline and inject only a minute amount. If this occurs, time and massage help to resolve it.

removing a mole or beauty mark

Contrary to widespread belief, moles and beauty marks—known as nevi to the medical profession—are not present at birth but develop over time, fueled by sun exposure during childhood and early adulthood. The average adult has up to forty nevi that gradually disappear with advancing age, but anyone with fifty to one hundred moles or more may be at greater than average risk for developing malignant melanoma and should be checked regularly by a dermatologist. Evenly colored moles are usually harmless, but it is sometimes hard for the untrained eye to distinguish a "typical" mole from a precancerous one. An atypical mole, also called a dysplastic nevus, may be a precursor of malignant melanoma and is often asymmetrical in shape with an irregular border, multiple colors, or a diameter that is bigger than a pencil eraser.

If you don't consider your "beauty mark" as beautiful as Cindy Crawford's or Niki Taylor's, it can be removed in a safe, simple lunchtime procedure. Laser surgery is not recommended for atypical nevi because removing only the superficial pigment may leave an actual or potential malignancy undiagnosed and untreated. Therefore, after the area has been numbed with an injection of lidocaine, unwanted beauty marks are typically removed with a scalpel, particularly if they're large and have protruding hair. The resulting wound may require tiny sutures that are covered with a small Band-Aid and removed in about a week. In some cases, the scalpel is held tangentially, parallel to the surface of the skin, and the mole is shaved down to the level of the skin, leaving the "roots" of the mole still present. This often results in a better cosmetic outcome, but there may be residual pigmentation at the site that appears as a flat brown freckle that can be lightened by gentle freezing or lasering or easily covered with foundation makeup. Whenever a mole or any growth is removed, the tissue is sent to a laboratory for a biopsy to ensure that it is benign.

removing skin tags

These common fleshy growths on the neck, under the arms, and in the inner thighs tend to run in families and are more common in overweight people. Sometimes the tags itch, especially when you're perspiring, and necklaces can get caught in the tags in the neck area. While it is not a medical necessity to remove skin tags, most people find them cosmetically unattractive and also annoying. Numerous tags—up to twenty or thirty—can be snipped off with scissors in one session or frozen with liquid nitrogen or lightly burned with an electrodesiccating machine in a matter of minutes. To numb the areas, EMLA cream is applied about an hour before your lunch break, or the doctor may inject the area with lidocaine immediately before the procedure. After a number of skin tags are removed, there may be tiny pinpoint scabs that can be covered immediately by makeup. In a week or two, the areas treated will be fully healed and smooth. Skin tags are so easy to remove in a "vanity session" with your dermatologist that satisfaction is all but guaranteed!

removing seborrheic keratoses

These light tan to dark brown "barnacles of life" that appear to be stuck onto the surface of the skin tend to run in families and are commonly seen in people as they age. The good news is that they can be easily scraped off with a curette, burned off with an electrocautery needle, frozen with liquid nitrogen, or vaporized with a CO_2 or erbium:YAG laser. If they are scraped, there is typically some mild bleeding that can be stemmed by the application of aluminum chloride. Antibiotic ointment and a small Band-Aid are all it takes for anyone to go back to work after this ideal lunchtime procedure. After a week or two, the skin fully heals, but there may be temporary discoloration that eventually disappears with no telltale scars.

removing tiny skin bumps

Small entirely benign facial skin growths are easily frozen, zapped with a laser or an electrocautery needle, or treated with acid. This is a blessing for people who have found that camouflage makeup doesn't hide what look like pimples under the skin but really aren't. Today, the self-consciousness about these tiny growths has been all but banished with treatments that get rid of dozens of them in as little as ten minutes. While most miscellaneous skin growths respond to treatment, portions of them may be located too deeply in the dermis to be reached safely by any method, hence the chance of recurrence.

These skin nuisances, with their intimidating medicalese names, include:

- Sebaceous hyperplasia: an overgrowth of sebaceous glands on the face, especially on the forehead

- Xanthelasma: yellowish deposits around the eye that may be a sign of high lipids, or triglycerides, in the blood
- Syringomas: tiny bumps derived from sweat glands under the eyes
- Trichoepitheliomas, angiofibromas, and hydrocystomas: little bumps around the sides of the nose
- Milia: tiny white bumps under the skin from clogged pores, which are commonly extracted with a special instrument

treating white scars or patches

Vitiligo, an autoimmune disease that runs in families, is a condition in which the body attacks its own pigment cells and leaves the skin mottled with stark white spots or widespread white patches. The condition is of unknown etiology and particularly devastating to dark-skinned people. Common treatments have always been cover-up makeup to hide the spots and ultraviolet light treatments to try to repigment them. But after the many ultraviolet light treatments that are necessary (sometimes more than one hundred), patients run a higher risk for developing squamous cell carcinoma and malignant melanoma years down the road.

Enter the new exciting excimer laser. After six to fourteen treatments, the ultraviolet laser beam that targets the white patches, while sparing the surrounding normal skin, yields visible results. While the treatment is not always successful, for some people it is the miracle they've been looking for. The excimer laser used for vitiligo (X Trac) is different from the excimer laser used by ophthalmologists in the LASIK procedure to reshape the eyeball and correct nearsightedness and farsightedness. The FDA has cleared the excimer laser not only for vitiligo but also for psoriasis, a chronic, inflammatory skin disorder (see Chapter 14, "Laser

Treatment of Red Problems"). The FDA has not yet approved the excimer laser for the treatment of flat white scars, but many doctors are encouraged by preliminary studies, believing it may hold promise for this purpose.

correcting deep ice-pick acne scars and depressed chicken pox scars

It's hard to describe the silent grief that people experience when their faces are marred by the scars of acne and their bodies with leftover chicken pox scars. Hear ye, hear ye: Suffer no more! After the area around your scar is numbed with lidocaine, the scar is excised with a scalpel or with a punch instrument that looks like a small cookie cutter, and the healthy skin on either side of the incision is stitched together. The most pitted or depressed scars can be filled in with grafts of skin from behind the ear, a procedure that is analogous to spackling a wall that will later be sanded and painted. Sometimes the grafts are sutured or glued into place. In about four to six weeks, after the grafts fully heal, the skin is gently buffed with a resurfacing laser or electric needle. Cover-up makeup then conceals a smooth skin surface and not an indented or bumpy one. It is possible to have a few tiny skin grafts placed during a lunch break.

correcting shallow indented scars

In a technique called subcision, the fibrous bands that anchor a depressed scar are severed, releasing the scar tissue and elevating the depression. There may be swelling and bruising at the site that are easily covered by makeup. Several sessions at one-month intervals may be necessary for optimal results. In addition, shallow, saucer-shaped scars can be treated with filling agents (see Chapter 6, "Getting Glamorous with Collagen Shots"), microdermabrasion (see Chapter 9, "Rejuvenating Your Skin with a Power Peel"), nonablative laser resurfacing (see Chapter 12, "Nonablative Lasers for Wrinkles"), and ablative laser resurfacing (see Chapter 16, "Not-So-Instant Beauty").

There are numerous other quick fixes—some covered by insurance—that include the treatment of precancerous actinic or solar keratoses, treatment of warts, and excision of small lumps and bumps like cysts and lipomas.

With today's "instant" procedures, there is no longer any reason to suffer with or be embarrassed by unattractive "thingies" on your skin. A few minutes at the dermatologist's office during your lunch break can fix so many of those little things that bother you a lot.

part two

a more fabulous-looking you!

getting glamorous with collagen shots

filling in wrinkles, plumping up indented scars, and enhancing thin lips

You can have a simple lunchtime "filling" that contains no calories, fats, or carbs. While millions of people have availed themselves of these quick fixes, no one could have been a more unlikely candidate than Thea, owner of a health-food store in northern California. The earthy forty-six-year-old seemed to embody everything that was desirable about the "natural" lifestyle and to have contempt for everything that was "unnatural."

For decades, this mother of two grown children and two teenagers cited herself as the best example of the products she sold: herbal potions that kept her skin amazingly young, vitamin-enriched shampoos that kept her long, tumbling hair shiny, and a vegetarian diet that kept her energy at peak level.

But Thea, who was a secret smoker and never pushed away a glass—or a bottle—of wine, started noticing in her early forties, at just about the same time she and her husband divorced, that her lips looked thinner and pinched, the "smoker's" lines around her mouth were deeper, and the nasolabial fold lines that ran from the sides of her nose to the corners of her mouth looked like crevasses. She hated the way she looked, and the stress of her life made her uncharacteristically moody. For the first time she could remember, she didn't have "all the answers."

But her friend Connie did. "Time may be a great healer," she told Thea, "but it's a lousy beautician!" First, she insisted that Thea highlight her hair, which the aging hippie loved. Then she insisted that Thea learn yoga, which she also loved. But the turning point came in 1996 when Connie insisted that the two of them go to the movies to see *The First Wives Club*. Thea roared and cheered when Goldie Hawn had collagen injected into her lips, but she was most struck by how young the actress looked, even though she knew the ditzy blonde was in the neighborhood of the big five-o when the movie was made.

It took two years for Thea the vegetarian to get past the fact that the collagen used in cosmetic procedures comes from cows, but once she tried it, she was as hooked on the glamour shots as she had become on highlighting her hair.

questions and answers about collagen

WHAT IS COLLAGEN?

Collagen (from the Greek word *kolla*, meaning "glue") is the most abundant protein in the human body. It gives support and structure to skin, bones, ligaments, and other body parts. The form of collagen used as a filling agent for cosmetic enhancement (which received FDA approval in 1981) is made from highly purified bovine collagen obtained from the hides of cows. Backed by a history of twenty years of use in 1.9 million patients worldwide, it remains the gold standard of fillers.

There are three types of collagen. Zyderm I, which is injected just below the surface of the skin into the dermis, has a thin consistency and is effective for softening fine lines. Zyderm II, a more concentrated form of collagen, is used to correct deeper lines and acne scars. Zyplast, which is injected even more deeply into the subcutaneous tissues, is the thickest form of collagen and is effective for improving the deepest folds and wrinkles. Clinicians often layer collagen, placing a thicker agent first to build a foundation and then using a thinner agent to augment the treatment.

IS COLLAGEN DERIVED FROM COWS SAFE?

Since bovine spongiform encephalopathy (mad cow disease) has terrorized Europe, people are legitimately concerned about any product that comes from cows. McGhan Medical, the company that manufactures Zyderm and Zyplast, has emphasized that since the 1980s, all the cows from which their product is derived have been raised in a "closed herd" on an isolated California ranch, fed grain that is grown solely on the ranch and does not contain outside sources of animal protein, and monitored closely and slaughtered on the ranch's property. According to the Food and Drug Administration, mad cow disease has never been diagnosed in the United States.

WHO IS A CANDIDATE FOR COLLAGEN INJECTIONS?

Facial wrinkles and creases begin to appear as the natural aging process breaks down collagen and elastin fibers under the skin and as a lifetime of squinting, frowning, smoking, and smiling takes its toll. A natural candidate for collagen injections is anyone who wants to improve the appearance of furrows and worry lines on the forehead, crow's feet at the corners of the eyes, lipstick "bleed" lines or "smoker's" lines around the mouth, marionette lines at the sides of the mouth, prominent nasolabial folds that extend from the outer nostrils to the corners of the mouth, and contour depressions and facial scarring from acne or injury. And because lips tend to get thinner with age, it is also effective in plumping up the lips. However, if you have sagging jowls and deeply etched marionette lines, collagen is not a replacement for a facelift because it does not tighten the skin or reposition under-lying muscles or fat.

ARE THERE ANY DISQUALIFYING HEALTH CONSIDERATIONS OR RISKS?

Allergy is a major consideration. If you have a history of allergy to beef or to the anesthetic lidocaine (which is mixed in with the collagen), you are not a candidate for collagen injections. To test for allergy, the manufacturer of the most popular form of bovine collagen, Zyderm, recommends placing a small amount of colla-gen in the skin of the forearm and repeating the test two weeks to a month later. If the test is not performed, patients run the risk of developing welts and red bumps at each site where the collagen is injected, which may persist for several months. Approximately 3 percent of the population is allergic to collagen. In addition, anyone with an autoimmune or connective tissue disease, such as lupus or scleroderma, should not have collagen injections. Patients with connective tissue diseases may have an increased susceptibility to allergic reactions or a tendency to metabolize collagen too quickly.

HOW IS THE PROCEDURE PERFORMED?

About an hour before the treatment, EMLA cream is often applied to numb the areas to be injected. Ice packs help as well. Then, while you are in a reclining or upright position, the doctor uses a fine needle to inject the appropriate amount of collagen (which also contains a local anesthetic to further reduce discomfort) to "fill out" the lines and wrinkles or plump up depressed scars to the level of the surrounding skin. Often, the collagen is injected along the course of a wrinkle in a series of little pricks or in a thin stream that is threaded under the skin.

WILL I NEED ANESTHESIA?

No sedation or anesthesia is required. EMLA cream and ice packs can numb the area and syringes of Zyderm come already mixed with 0.3 percent of the local anesthetic lidocaine.

HOW WILL I LOOK IMMEDIATELY AFTER?

Your face will appear smoother, with fewer lines, wrinkles, and indented scars. You may have a few marks from the needle pricks, but they can easily be covered with makeup. There may be slight redness and also temporary tiny bumps where the skin was injected, which can be reduced by massage. Bruising occurs in less than 10 percent of patients but is not uncommon in those who are taking blood thinners like aspirin or Motrin. If you experience any swelling or bruising, an ice pack to the area will help. Occasionally, injected collagen may be visible as a white bump that is seen through the skin at the treatment site. This may persist for a few weeks to a few months. There may also be what doctors call a temporary "overcorrection," meaning that it may appear that you have gotten more collagen than you wanted. Fortunately, this is short-lived and dissipates within days.

HOW WILL I FEEL IMMEDIATELY AFTER?

Absolutely fine and able to return to work or play without hesitation. This is one procedure that truly requires absolutely no downtime.

HOW LONG DOES THE PROCEDURE TAKE?
Approximately fifteen to twenty minutes.

HOW MANY TREATMENTS WILL I REQUIRE
AND HOW LONG WILL THEY LAST?
Depending on the condition of your face, your age, and your
expectations, one to three syringes of collagen may be injected at
the first treatment session. In some cases, additional filling sessions are necessary at two-week intervals until the desired cosmetic result is achieved. Since the body metabolizes bovine
collagen, the results last for only about three months. New collagen must be injected about four times a year to maintain your
new look. The treatment of acne scars tends to last longer. In rare
cases, the injections seem to stimulate the body's own production of collagen, and improvement lasts for more than a year.

WHAT IS THE BEST TIME TO HAVE
COLLAGEN INJECTIONS?
Lunchtime is perfect since the procedure only takes fifteen to
twenty minutes and yields immediate results. But if you have a
special occasion planned, schedule the treatment one to two
weeks ahead to make sure that any minor bruising from the needle pricks is completely gone.

CAN COLLAGEN INJECTIONS BE COMBINED
WITH OTHER PROCEDURES DURING THE SAME
TREATMENT SESSION?
While collagen injections are often combined with a number of
cosmetic procedures, collagen is most commonly administered
with Botox injections (see Chapter 7, "Looking Younger with
Botox Shots"). Like soup and sandwich, they go together! Colla-

common sites for collagen and other fillers

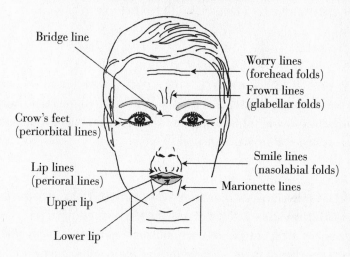

Bridge line

Worry lines
(forehead folds)

Frown lines
(glabellar folds)

Crow's feet
(periorbital lines)

Lip lines
(perioral lines)

Smile lines
(nasolabial folds)

Marionette lines

Upper lip

Lower lip

gen is thought of as an adjunct to Botox and vice versa. Collagen is mainly used to plump up lips and fill in the wrinkles on the *lower* half of the face, and Botox is infinitely superior for eradicating wrinkles on the *upper* half of the face and around the eyes.

WHAT SPECIAL TRAINING IS REQUIRED TO ADMINISTER COLLAGEN INJECTIONS?

Board-certified dermatologists or plastic surgeons are specially trained to perform cosmetic procedures that involve filling agents and the placement of needles. In some states, however, physicians' assistants, nurse practitioners, and registered nurses are allowed to administer collagen injections. But do your homework! Collagen and Botox injections—into your face!—require both skill and art, and some practitioners are simply better than others. In all cases, it is imperative that a strict standard of sterility is adhered to and that the facility meets all safety standards established by the Occupational Safety and Health Administration (see Chapter 4, "Better Safe Than Sorry").

WILL PEOPLE BE ABLE TO TELL THAT I HAVE HAD A PROCEDURE DONE?

The effects are subtle, but most people will tell you that your skin looks wonderful, smooth, and youthful, and that you appear well rested and revitalized.

ARE THERE ANY COMPLICATIONS ASSOCIATED WITH COLLAGEN INJECTIONS?

Most people experience no complications. In the rare event of an allergic reaction in the face, which occurs in approximately four out of ten thousand patients—even, rarely, in those who have passed the preprocedure skin test—there may be constant or intermittent swelling, itching, firmness at the site, and red bumps that can last up to nine months or more. There may also be painful cystic abscesses that need to be drained. Sometimes Kenalog, a steroid, is injected into the area to decrease the inflammation. Those who have a history of cold sores are often prescribed an antiviral medication before collagen injections since they run the risk of developing an outbreak at the site.

WHAT DO COLLAGEN INJECTIONS COST?

While the rates vary, depending on the area of the country and the individual physician, treatment cost depends on how many vials of collagen are used during the procedure. The average cost is approximately $500 to $600 for one vial (approximately 1 cc) of collagen. Usually one to three vials are injected during a single treatment session.

WHAT IMPROVEMENT CAN I
REASONABLY EXPECT?

If your skin is sun-damaged or has very deep wrinkles, you may
be disappointed with collagen injections. But if you understand
that the results of collagen treatments are subtle and last only
about three months, you will be very pleased with the degree to
which they effectively eliminate or significantly diminish bothersome fine lines and other signs of aging. The key to satisfaction
with any procedure is realistic expectations. In other words, if
you're fifty and expect to look thirty after collagen treatments,
you'll be disappointed. Realistically, however, you can expect to
look like a terrific forty-something-year-old!

WHAT QUESTIONS SHOULD I
ASK MY PHYSICIAN?

- How much experience have you had administering collagen
  injections?
- Have your patients had any complications from collagen?
  What were they?
- Can I speak to any of your patients who have had collagen?
- How many vials of collagen or how many treatment sessions
  will I need for optimal results?

ARE THERE ALTERNATIVE FILLING
AGENTS TO ZYDERM AND ZYPLAST?

While the perfect filling agent has not yet been developed, a
number of alternatives offer advantages over Zyderm and
Zyplast in certain circumstances. Despite manufacturers' claims
that this or that filler lasts longer than the competition's, most
fillers are temporary, lasting only three to four months.

Autologen is custom-made collagen that is extracted and
purified from remnants of your own skin during a previous

facelift or tummy tuck and injected at a later time. This option exists for anyone who is allergic to bovine (cow) collagen.

Dermalogen, another form of collagen that can be injected, is derived from the donated skin of human cadavers. After rigorous screening—including the donors' medical records, cause of death, social history, and negative findings for syphilis, hepatitis B and C, and HIV—the collagen is treated with powerful antiviral agents before being processed into Dermalogen. The entire process is overseen by the American Association of Tissue Banks, which is regulated by the FDA. No skin test is required for Dermalogen because allergic reactions are not known to occur with human collagen. Unlike bovine collagen, Dermalogen is not premixed with lidocaine and therefore the treatment is more uncomfortable, although EMLA cream and ice packs that are applied before the treatment significantly diminish any discomfort.

CosmoDerm is the first collagen product to be created from a single cell of a male infant's foreskin by the process of bioengineering. The newest filling agent on the cosmetic-enhancement block, it is not yet known how long its effects will last. Maureen Dowd, a *New York Times* columnist, reported that, incredibly, "the foreskin of one infant boy may be bioengineered into a supply that will replicate endlessly, providing plumped-up lips, etc., for women all over the world, ad infinitum. A bris to remember!"

Cymetra is derived from the processed skin of human cadavers and so recipients do not require allergy testing. The material, which is screened rigorously and treated with antiviral agents, is usually injected into subcutaneous tissue with a slightly larger needle than is used for other filling procedures.

Isologen derives from the collagen-producing cells of human skin from behind the ear, which is grown in test tubes. When the cells are injected into wrinkles, they fill in lines and also produce new collagen strands that promise to prevent wrinkles from returning.

Fibrel is a gelatin-based filler that combines pig protein with your own serum. A simple skin test can also detect allergy. In the procedure, a tube of your blood is withdrawn and processed to separate the red blood cells from the serum. The gelatin is then diluted with some of your own serum and injected to fill in wrinkles and acne scars. *Note: Jewish women who are kosher or Muslim women who also eschew pork are advised to tell their doctors of their beliefs before being injected with Fibrel.*

Silicone was developed in the 1930s and first used for tissue augmentation in 1965. But when adulterated (or impure) forms of silicone were injected into the skin, numerous disastrous complications resulted and the agent fell into disrepute after reports cited foreign body reactions, migration to other parts of the body, and implication in autoimmune diseases. Recently, two silicone products, AdatoSil 5000 and Silikone 1000, were introduced to the ophthalmology market to help repair detached retinas. Some dermatologists have been injecting these agents into the skin for "off-label" cosmetic purposes. Silicone is now being investigated for use as a permanent filling agent under the name SilSkin. If approved by the FDA, it may signal a rebirth of silicone in soft-tissue augmentation.

Fascian is derived from human tissue that is freeze-dried, irradiated, and stored in tissue banks. Packaged in prefilled syringes, it is rehydrated with saline or lidocaine and injected into the lips, nasolabial folds, and cheeks. But questions remain about the ability of the product to replace the body's own collagen and, more important, about the possibility that human DNA may linger in the processed material and therefore have the potential to transmit diseases.

Human fat was first used for tissue augmentation more than a hundred years ago. When it is carefully removed from soft-tissue areas like the thighs, buttocks, knees, and abdomen and injected into the tops of the hands, depressions around the temples, under the eyes, in the cheek hollows, and around the mouth, chin, and lips, long-lasting and often permanent results can be achieved. Most doctors prefer using fresh fat for lipo-transfer, extracting it from the belly, buttocks, or thighs with a small syringe and then immediately injecting it into the face. Some doctors harvest the fat and flash-freeze it for future use, but the jury is still out about the degree to which fat cells remain viable after freezing and defrosting. When your own fat is used as filler, there is no chance of allergy, immune reaction, or rejection. Often, the fat is molded and shaped by external manual massage after implantation. Since a larger needle is used in this procedure, bruising is more common. But it can still be a lunchtime procedure if small quantities are injected.

Hylaform Gel, a form of hyaluronic acid (a polysaccharide that is found in skin cells), is derived from the combs of roosters and used throughout the world for facial augmentation, especially to plump up lips, but it is currently not licensed in the United States. The fact that no skin test is necessary provides an advantage over bovine collagen. The Hylaform substance attracts water molecules, so lips stay nice and full, but not overly puffy. Restylane, another hyaluronic acid, is derived from streptococcal bacteria, marketed in a prefilled syringe, and injected in a linear, threadlike stream. Restylane-Fine Line is injected with a tiny needle into very fine lines, and Perlane, a more robust form, is used for deeper wrinkles. Clinical trials of Restylane are currently being conducted in the United States. Temporary reactions to these agents include redness, bruising, and acne, and, in the case of Hylaform Gel, some cases of prolonged swelling.

Artecoll combines bovine collagen with synthetic beads of Plexiglas. Doctors use the collagen as a vehicle for implanting the beads in the body to fill in deep wrinkles and furrows. While the collagen is metabolized, the beads remain. The filling-in effect ostensibly works when the body's natural formation of collagen surrounds the beads, providing a long-lasting if not permanent filling-in effect. Patients must have skin tests for allergy prior to receiving Artecoll. This agent has been used safely and effectively in Canada, Europe, Mexico, and South America since 1993. It is currently being investigated but is not yet available in the United States.

The following implants are placed in the skin with a minor surgical procedure. They are used as filling agents but must be implanted rather than injected. While these procedures can be performed during a lunch break, the temporary swelling that often follows may make you want to call it a day.

Gore-Tex, a synthetic substance used to make ski jackets, is threaded under the skin to rebuild thin lips and to elevate wrinkles from below. Since the substance is not absorbed, the results are permanent. But sometimes the threads extrude, causing them to protrude at the injection site, or the implant shifts under the skin and has to be removed.

SoftForm is a tube-shaped implant made from the same material as Gore-Tex and used for the same cosmetic enhancements. Because of its hollow shape, skin grows through the tube, anchoring it in place. The implant can be permanent, or it can be removed at a future date since the skin does not adhere to its nonstick surface. To make lips appear larger, a local anesthetic is usually administered before SoftForm is threaded through a tiny incision in the corner of the mouth and around the lips to the opposite corner. Or it can be threaded under the nasolabial folds to build them up and decrease their depth. Tiny stitches are needed where the implant enters and exits the skin. UltraSoft, a new softer, more pliable version of SoftForm, claims to provide results that are more natural than its predecessor.

Alloderm comes from the skin of human cadavers and is treated chemically to remove cellular components that might cause rejection. It is derived from the same source as Cymetra, but Cymetra can be injected whereas Alloderm comes in sheets that are rolled and placed in the lips through small incisions, resulting in fuller lips. Originally, Alloderm was touted as being permanent, but clinical experience has shown that over a year or two it usually dissipates or is absorbed by the body.

Dermaplant, an Alloderm-like material produced by the manufacturers of Dermalogen, comes from the dermis of human cadavers and is implanted in much the same way as Alloderm.

WHAT IS THE SATISFACTION RATE FROM COLLAGEN AND OTHER FILLER INJECTIONS?

While no perfect, completely natural, or permanent filling agent yet exists, most people are delighted with the relatively short "fix" that collagen injections and other fillers afford them in terms of looking younger, getting rid of unwanted lines, and generally feeling rejuvenated.

looking younger with Botox shots

relaxing the muscles that cause wrinkles, worry lines, frown lines, and crow's feet

Finally, a day off from your hectic life! What to do? For one thing, you can treat yourself to a lunch break that is leisurely, unrushed, and downright self-indulgent. Stroll the mall, try on this or that bauble or outfit, or treat yourself to a massage. Ah, what a wonderful fantasy!

But it doesn't have to be a fantasy when it comes to relaxing—even banishing—your wrinkles, worry lines, frown lines, and crow's feet. That's what Dorothy, a forty-eight-year-old special-education teacher, finally determined to do when it dawned on her that the wedding she had spent so much time planning for her only daughter was less than a month away and that the flowers, cake, invitations, menu, and every other detail had been attended to—but not herself!

While she had managed to find the time to buy a beautiful dress and, for her, atypically glamorous shoes, the problem, she said, was "the rest of me." Always attractive but never particularly vain, Dorothy began to look at herself in the mirror in a new way, stretching out the horizontal lines on her forehead and on the bridge of her nose "to see how I'd look without wrinkles" and even "practicing" smiling without squinting her eyes to see if she could do away with the pesky crow's feet that crinkled up every time she smiled or laughed.

Makeup didn't work but just caked and collected in the lines of Dorothy's face. She had all but resigned herself to hiding behind her bangs or "looking my age" when her daughter came to the rescue. "That's so retro, Mom," the bride-to-be announced. "Go for Botox and get gorgeous fast!"

The idea of going to a doctor for what she called a "vanity treatment" was alien and even frightening to Dorothy. But after a week of nagging by her daughter and after thinking about how old she might look in the wedding pictures, she relented, learning everything she could about Botox injections and, at last, taking a lunch break to "get gorgeous fast." At the wedding, she danced the night away, looking more like her daughter's sister than her mother!

questions and answers about Botox

WHAT IS BOTOX?

Botox is the trade name for a purified version of botulinum toxin type A, a nerve impulse blocker produced by bacteria. For cosmetic purposes, it is injected in minuscule amounts into specific muscles. It binds to the endings of nerves and prevents the release of chemical transmitters that activate the muscles under the skin. Botox injections *temporarily* weaken and relax these muscles, thus reducing the wrinkles that are produced by habitual muscular contractions. The procedure—which essentially achieves the same result as a surgical brow lift—is most effective in the upper part of the face, specifically in targeting crow's feet, worry lines on the forehead, and the frown lines that result from the gathering or knitting of skin tissue into folds or furrows between the eyebrows.

The repeated—and unconscious—action of the underlying muscles associated with smiling, squinting, and frowning leave deep wrinkles, which often give people an angry, stressed, or perturbed look that is at odds with the way they actually feel. Once the muscle is injected with Botox, it relaxes, and it becomes impossible to make a formerly undesirable facial expression.

Botox has been used safely and effectively for more than twenty years in the treatment of a number of noncosmetic medical conditions, most notably to correct amblyopia ("lazy eye" or crossed eyes) by injection into the extraocular muscles of children, and blepharospasm (uncontrollable tics or twitches of the eyelid). Like a number of medications that were approved by the Food and Drug Administration for specific conditions—such as the muscle relaxant Miltown that was found to be a powerful tranquilizer and the acne medicine Retin-A that was found to reduce fine lines in the face—Botox, too, proved to have valuable off-label uses. The FDA approved Botox for cosmetic procedures in early 2002.

The versatility of Botox was originally demonstrated by an unanticipated, indeed serendipitous, observation in 1987, when Canadian ophthalmologist Jean Carruthers noticed that when she injected Botox to correct a patient's eye problem, the fine lines and wrinkles on the same side of the forehead disappeared. She and her husband, dermatologist Alastair R. Carruthers, soon began using the toxin for cosmetic purposes—to their patients' everlasting delight. But it took another decade for Botox injections to become wildly popular. Today they are considered extremely safe all over the world. In fact, they were the most sought after cosmetic procedure performed in the United States in 2000. European doctors primarily use Dysport, a product also made from the botulinum toxin type A.

While Botox has officially been FDA-cleared for the purpose of injecting vertical frown lines between the eyebrows, it is also commonly used to treat:

- Horizontal lines on the bridge of the nose
- Squint lines or crow's feet at the outer corners of the eyes
- Horizontal worry lines on the forehead
- Platysmal muscle bands or neck cords ("turkey neck")
- Elevation of the brow for a more youthful appearance

WHO IS A CANDIDATE?

Anyone who has frown lines, worry lines, or crow's feet and is not ready for a surgical brow lift but wants a "quick fix."

ARE THERE HEALTH CONSIDERATIONS THAT WOULD DISQUALIFY ME OR INCREASE MY RISKS FOR THIS PROCEDURE?

Women who are pregnant or breast-feeding should not have Botox injections because it is not known if there are any long-term effects on or any possibility of absorption by the developing baby. People who have neuromuscular diseases such as myasthenia gravis and amyotrophic lateral sclerosis (Lou Gehrig's disease) should not have Botox injections because of a risk of exacerbating the disease, nor should those with known allergies to human albumin (which is contained in the Botox preparation). In addition, anyone taking a blood-thinning medication such as Coumadin should consult with his or her doctor before having Botox because of the increased risk of bruising from the needle injections.

ARE THERE ANY ADDITIONAL RISKS?

Occasionally, a small subcutaneous bruise known as a hematoma arises where the needle was inserted. If Botox is injected into a muscle group for which it was not intended, there might be a drooping of the eyelid (eyelid ptosis) or eyebrow (brow ptosis), which can be alleviated with over-the-counter or prescription eye drops. Fortunately, these side effects don't last more than a week or two. Rarely, there may be complaints of headache, dry eyes, double vision, sensitivity to light, or an overproduction of tears in the eyes, which are always temporary. But risk factors, no matter how small, are still risk factors, which is why you should discuss them thoroughly with your doctor *before* the procedure. In addition, it is wise to avoid having this procedure performed in a spa or salon. Instead, seek out a board-certified dermatologist or plastic surgeon with an in-depth knowledge of facial anatomy and a lot of experience in administering Botox injections. (See Chapter 4, "Better Safe Than Sorry.")

ARE THERE ALTERNATIVES TO THE PROCEDURE?

A surgical brow lift provides a permanent solution to furrowing and wrinkling by removing the same muscles that Botox only relaxes temporarily. To deal with crow's feet, some people opt for laser resurfacing or a chemical peel, which provide less improvement than is achieved by Botox shots because the muscles around the eyes still contract, producing the dynamic wrinkles that appear each time you smile or squint.

HOW DO I PREPARE FOR MY
BOTOX PROCEDURE?

There is very little preparation. Sometimes, your doctor will prescribe EMLA, a topical anesthetic cream containing lidocaine
and prilocaine, that you can apply an hour before the treatment
to numb the areas to be injected with Botox. Also, placing ice on
the areas immediately before injection will increase the numbness and reduce any possible discomfort.

If you tend to bruise easily, it's a good idea to discontinue
taking aspirin or any nonsteroidal anti-inflammatory medication
several days before the procedure, always under the supervision
of your doctor.

WHAT ARE THE TIMING OPTIONS
FOR THIS PROCEDURE?

Botox injections are the premier lunchtime procedure! But if
you have a special occasion coming up, it's best to have the
injections a week or two in advance in order to give the Botox
time to kick in and avoid any possible welts or bruises. Usually the full effect of the treatment is realized in about five
days.

HOW IS THE PROCEDURE PERFORMED?

Using a microneedle, a tiny amount of Botox is injected very precisely into several anatomical locations on the face. Because the
needle is so fine and only a small amount of liquid is used, discomfort is short-lived, most patients comparing the injections to
bug bites. Some doctors use an electromyography machine
(EMG) to help locate the specific muscle to be injected. The
device, similar to a Geiger counter, translates the activity of the
muscle into a sound. After the doctor places the needle into
the muscle that lies between the eyebrows, he or she asks the

common sites for Botox

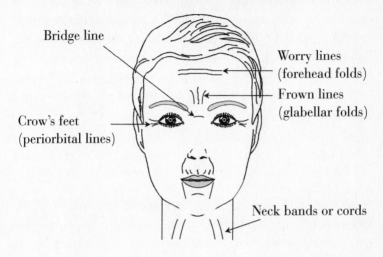

Bridge line

Worry lines
(forehead folds)

Frown lines
(glabellar folds)

Crow's feet
(periorbital lines)

Neck bands or cords

patient to frown. If the needle is in the right spot, the EMG machine increases in volume, indicating that the correct muscle has been located.

HOW MANY TREATMENTS WILL I REQUIRE?
In about 80 percent of cases, only one treatment is required. While the first session usually yields excellent results, some patients return for a touch-up treatment about two weeks after their first Botox session.

CAN THIS PROCEDURE BE COMBINED WITH OTHER PROCEDURES ON THE SAME DAY?
Botox injections that are administered primarily to the upper part of the face are often combined with injections of collagen that are primarily used on the wrinkles in the lower areas of the face.

WILL I NEED AN ANESTHETIC?

No sedation or anesthesia is required—just an ice pack. For people who are very sensitive, EMLA topical numbing cream can be applied to the treated areas about an hour before the treatment to take the edge off any uncomfortable sensation from the needle. There may be a temporary twinge with each injection, but the final result is so thrilling that any discomfort is soon forgotten.

IS ANY SPECIAL TRAINING REQUIRED TO ADMINISTER BOTOX?

A precise understanding of the anatomy of the muscles of the face is paramount in ensuring a safe procedure. While no special training is required, increasing numbers of dermatologists and plastic surgeons are now responding to the demand for Botox injections by learning the technique from one another.

HOW LONG DOES THE PROCEDURE TAKE?

Botox injections are one of the fastest cosmetic treatments in medical history, usually lasting only five or ten minutes for the entire upper half of the face. Injections into the lower neck area take a little longer.

HOW WILL I LOOK IMMEDIATELY AFTER?

Actually, the same as you looked before the treatment because it takes a few days for the Botox to work its magic. There are usually no telltale signs of what you've been up to on your lunch break, so no one has to know. However, sometimes a few tiny needle marks may be visible on your face and you may have some temporary bruising at one or two injection sites. If your doctor inadvertently hits a blood vessel that causes your skin to become slightly reddened, swollen, or bruised, the area can be easily covered with camouflage makeup. Placing an ice pack on the skin and applying pressure immediately after Botox injections helps to minimize any bruising or welting.

HOW WILL I FEEL IMMEDIATELY AFTER?
You will feel absolutely fine and be able to go right back to whatever you were doing before.

WHAT DOES THE RECOVERY ENTAIL?
Do not lie down or take a nap for approximately four hours after your Botox treatment. If you have to pick up something from the floor, bend at the knees with your head upright. This will ensure that the Botox stays in the muscles for which it was intended and does not drift to other muscles.

If the area between your eyebrows was injected, make a conscious attempt to frown during the first several hours after the injection. If your forehead was injected, raise your eyebrows often. And if the crow's feet around your eyes were injected, try to squint during that same time period. This helps the muscles to soak up the Botox, allowing it to kick in more quickly.

Do not massage any areas that were injected to avoid inadvertent migration of the Botox to surrounding muscles.

To reduce any swelling, an ice pack is helpful. To cover any bruising, use camouflage makeup.

HOW LONG DOES IT TAKE BEFORE I CAN RETURN TO NORMAL ACTIVITY?
You can drive yourself home or back to work immediately, but refrain from any strenuous activities and aerobic exercises until the following day.

WILL PEOPLE BE ABLE TO TELL THAT I HAVE HAD SOMETHING DONE?

While Botox injections don't tighten sagging skin, they can nevertheless make a very dramatic change in your appearance. Within a few days, the wrinkles that you're accustomed to seeing—and hating—every time you look in the mirror will either be totally gone or significantly diminished. Your family, friends, and colleagues will undoubtedly tell you that you never looked better. And don't be surprised if you take every opportunity to look in the mirror just to admire your new, quite fabulous look.

WHAT CAN I REASONABLY EXPECT?

Botox injections will smooth away "dynamic" wrinkles—the kind you get from the contractions of underlying facial muscles—and give you a more youthful appearance. But they cannot reverse sun damage or tighten loose skin that sags as a result of chronological aging since these changes are not solely related to the muscles of facial expression.

HOW LONG WILL THE RESULTS LAST?

Botox injections are a *temporary* solution that lasts from three to six months; follow-up treatments are usually performed two to four times a year. Clinical studies have shown that the effect increases over time and that people who have had multiple treatments seem to require injections less frequently, possibly because the injected muscles undergo a slight degree of atrophy.

WHAT IS THE SATISFACTION RATE FROM THIS PROCEDURE?

Extremely high! Many women prefer to save up money for their Botox treatments rather than buy a new outfit. "A dress can be worn only a few times," one woman remarked, "but you wear

your face every day." When people have their first Botox injections, the results are so dramatic and the satisfaction level so
great that they seem to be hooked for life. This "addiction" has
become so popular that many women consider it as necessary as
getting their hair colored. Indeed, it is not uncommon for a
woman planning to attend a special event to have a manicure,
pedicure, waxing, highlights, *and* Botox all in one day. In fact,
according to numerous news reports, plastic surgeons in Bev-
erly Hills ran out of Botox during Academy Awards week!

WHAT ARE THE MOST COMMON ANXIETIES ABOUT BOTOX INJECTIONS?

Some patients fear the procedure because they associate botulinum with the very real fear of botulism. When the toxin is
found in contaminated food and ingested orally, it can cause generalized paralysis that leads to death. This fear, however, is
unfounded with injections because Botox is perfectly safe when
minute amounts are injected into a specific muscle and not
ingested. Others worry about looking "plastic," "masklike," or
"unnatural," or losing the ability to express facial emotion. In
fact, Botox does not paralyze or freeze muscles *permanently* but
rather weakens and relaxes them *temporarily*, giving the face a
smooth and natural look.

Another anxiety is that Botox will cause a generalized numbing sensation. In fact, it interferes only with the movement of the
muscle and not with any sensation—touching, tickling, stroking,
and the like—in the overlying skin. Some people fear that the
muscle that is treated will atrophy, which is now believed to be a
welcome effect that may serve to lessen the number of treatments
needed over a lifetime.

Another fear is of an allergic reaction, but there has *never*
been a report of an allergic or anaphylactic reaction.

Fear of needles is also a reason people pass on the procedure. While the topical EMLA cream numbs the area, it does

nothing to ease the mind of the needle-phobic patient. The solution to this phobia always lies with the ability of the physician and his or her staff to create a calming atmosphere and some distracting chatter.

Finally, some people are afraid that they will develop antibodies to Botox that will cause their system to reject it. On the rare occasion that this occurs, the only effect is that the injections will no longer work as well. Currently, newer substances are being developed. One that is already marketed commercially is botulinum toxin type B, or Myobloc, which differs from Botox in several ways.

For instance, once Botox is shipped from the manufacturer, it must be kept frozen in the doctor's office and, once defrosted, used either the same day or over the ensuing week, after which it loses some of its potency. In contrast, Myobloc is stable at room temperature for six months and usable for eighteen months when refrigerated. Additionally, Myobloc has proved to be a boon to the small but growing number of people who have become immune to Botox after large-volume injections into the neck area. Like Botox, Myobloc's line-eradicating effects last about three to six months, but it is reportedly more painful than Botox because it contains an acidic preservative that can cause a stinging sensation. Its most common side effect is temporary dry mouth.

WHAT DO BOTOX INJECTIONS COST?

While the fees vary, the average cost for Botox treatment is approximately $400 to $500 for each anatomical area. However pricey this seems, most people who have had the shots insist that Botox gave them the biggest bang for their buck!

WHAT QUESTIONS DO I NEED TO ASK MY DOCTOR?

- How much experience have you had administering Botox?
- Have you ever had complications with Botox? What were they?
- Can I speak with any of your patients who have had Botox injections?
- Will I be charged if I return for a touch-up treatment? (Touch-up treatments can be complimentary, at a lesser or reduced charge, or at the full charge once again. It is important to discuss these issues with your doctor before your treatment.)

WHAT OTHER CONDITIONS CAN BOTOX TREAT?

Profuse sweating (hyperhidrosis). A single treatment of Botox can alleviate the social and professional embarrassment of excessive sweating for months by treating the sweat glands of the skin. This involves injections directly into the skin under the arm, the palms of the hands or soles of the feet, and occasionally the scalp line. Injections can be repeated indefinitely once or twice a year to maintain dryness, but with repeated treatments some patients run the risk of developing antibodies that may render the treatment less effective. Traditionally, antiperspirants and topical agents containing skin-irritating ingredients like aluminum chloride have been used to combat this persistent condition, as well as the time-consuming iontophoresis, a technique in which an electric current is passed through a liquid bath and temporarily inhibits sweating of the palms or soles. But these treatments have been only moderately helpful and temporary.

In preparation, EMLA cream, a spray of topical anesthetic, or a simple nerve block numbs the palms, soles, or armpits. (Some doctors treat only one palm at a time.) Possible side effects may include temporary and localized muscle weakness or minor pain or stinging at the injection site. It usually takes a week for profuse sweating to decrease, and the effect lasts from six to ten months. The cost can be higher than facial treatments with Botox since larger quantities are needed to produce the desired effect.

"Turkey neck." Platysmal muscle bands (or cords) are often visible on the aging neck, creating that gobbledy-gobbledy look that has kept turtleneck sweaters, scarves, and multiple strands of pearls so popular for so long. "Turkey neck" can be treated with Botox on a lunch break, but with a caveat: It's important that you go to a doctor who is an expert in administering injections in the neck area, specifically into the platysmal cords and not the surrounding muscles to avoid side effects like a change in your voice or difficulty swallowing. The treatment will not get rid of any fat in the neck area, but the cords and bands will become less obvious. The good news is that in three to seven days after the treatment you'll be able to put your turtleneck sweater in mothballs!

Lipstick "bleed" lines. Botox is sometimes used very carefully and in small amounts to diminish smile lines, creases, or lipstick "bleed" lines around the mouth. A tiny bit of Botox can inhibit contraction of the muscle around the mouth, giving the lip a much softer look. For this reason, Botox can be a wonderful adjunct to collagen or other filling agents. However, the muscle around the mouth is needed not only for smiling but also for important functions like sipping, eating, and kissing. Therefore, relaxing or weakening this muscle too much might result in drooling and difficulty in eating, drinking, or speaking.

Gummy smile. For people who don't like the amount of upper gum their smiles reveal, Botox can provide subtle but satisfying results. During treatment, the patient is asked to smile as broadly as possible in order to reveal the maximum amount of upper gum. Then the doctor injects Botox into the top portion of the nasolabial folds (the lines that run from the side of the nostrils to the corners of the mouth). When the underlying muscle is relaxed, the upper lip becomes slightly elongated, effectively covering the upper teeth and hiding the unwanted appearance of the gum when smiling broadly or laughing.

Drooping eyebrows. When injected into specific areas, Botox can elevate the outer corners of the eyebrows to give them a better arch, a more feminine look, and a more open-eyed appearance.

Migraine headaches. While Botox has not been FDA-approved for the treatment of migraines, relief from these intractably painful headaches (and from tension headaches as well) has been found to be a common side effect of the injections. So far, the reasons are unclear, but numerous women have reported that Botox shots not only made them look younger but also eliminated their migraines. "After my first treatment," one patient remarked, "my husband volunteered to pay for follow-ups. My headaches went away so even our sex life got better!"

feeling refreshed with chemical peels

glycolic acid and other superficial chemical peels that leave your skin silky smooth and bursting with youth

Danielle, a jet-setting buyer for an upscale catalog house in Chicago, met every Wednesday for lunch at Morton's with friends who were equally busy scaling the heights of their own professions. The waiters knew better than to ply the ladies with sizzling steaks and instead brought them "the usual"—mile-high salads of fresh vegetables, a round of cool, refreshing wine spritzers, and desserts of fresh fruit.

Much of their talk was personal, about the doctor's kids, the lawyer's political aspirations, the architect's exotic trips, the dot-com executive's job search, and Danielle's latest visit with her psychic. While the women were all between the ages of thirty-seven and forty-four, they never ended their hour-long luncheon without one or the other of them sharing the most recent "cure" she had either read about or tried to stem the encroaching ravages of age. During one of their get-togethers, Franca, the architect (whom the group considered their resident historian), couldn't wait to share everything she had recently learned about alpha hydroxy acids.

She told them that AHAs were "fruit acids" derived from

apples (malic acid), grapes (tartaric acid), sour milk (lactic acid), citrus fruits (citric acid), and sugarcane (glycolic acid). "In ancient times," she explained, "people somehow knew that when they bathed in milk or rubbed wine on their faces, they were exfoliating their skin and turning back the hands of time, just as my Italian grandmother must have known that using lemon juice on her face would lighten the discolorations."

The group's lunch hour was up. They made Franca promise to continue her "lecture" the following Wednesday. After the women had learned "everything they ever wanted to know" about AHAs, two of them ran to the drugstore for over-the-counter AHAs and two decided to have glycolic acid peels at their dermatologists' offices. Danielle postponed the treatment for a month because she said that her psychic told her "to focus on my business and not myself."

questions and answers about chemical peels

HOW DO AHAS WORK?

AHAs penetrate the skin's outer layer, peel away its horny cells, and deliver a uniform rosy glow. It's still not known whether or not they truly increase the production of collagen and improve the quality of elastic fibers in the skin. The effectiveness of an AHA depends primarily on its concentration and its pH (the measure of acidity). The lower the pH, the more acidic the product; the more acidic, the more irritating; the more irritating, the better it works! However, a number of doctors believe that buffered or neutralized AHAs are equally effective while causing less irritation.

For superficial peels, aestheticians in salons are allowed by the FDA to use up to 30 percent glycolic acid with a pH of 3.0. If an aesthetician administers a series of "refreshing" peels under the supervision of a physician, up to 70 percent glycolic acid may be applied with a pH that is even lower than 3.0.

Patients having a concentrated glycolic acid peel must be closely monitored because the longer the acid is left on the skin, the deeper the penetration and the greater the irritation.

WHAT IS THE CONTROVERSY ABOUT HAVING CHEMICAL PEELS IN A SPA OR SALON?

In many states, such as New York, glycolic acid peels may be performed by aestheticians who are trained in the procedure and use a glycolic acid concentration of not more than 30 percent with a pH of not less than 3.0. In other states, such as New Jersey, only medical doctors are allowed to administer glycolic acid peels, as it is considered "the practice of medicine." Many aestheticians insist that restricting their ability to perform the peels curtails their autonomy and incomes. While the licenses of aestheticians allow them to work on hair, nails, or the dead top layer of skin, chemical peels affect deeper, living tissues.

Doctors believe that minimally trained spa employees are not equipped to diagnose or treat the potential side effects of chemical peels such as wounds, burns, scarring, infections, or other complications. In a recent survey conducted by the American Society for Dermatologic Surgery, 45 percent of physicians reported increases in complications from chemical peels and other procedures performed by nonphysicians. Industry standards preclude nonphysicians from performing any procedures that go deeper than the skin's dead cell layers without physician supervision. But with chemical peels becoming more widely available, such standards are not always followed.

WHAT IS A GLYCOLIC ACID PEEL?

Glycolic acid, a type of AHA, has the lowest molecular weight of all fruit acids, which allows it to penetrate the skin so effectively that it brings about the most dramatic and beneficial changes of all the fruit acid peels. While this type of superficial peel is often referred to as "the lunchtime peel," it is more accurately described as skin "washing," "sloughing," "freshening," or "exfoliation." The acid loosens or dissolves the gluelike bonds or cellular cement that characterizes skin conditions like acne, sun damage, and hyperpigmentation, lifting the dead cells of the stratum corneum without wounding the skin. The effect is similar to removing the dried-out upper layer of an onion's skin to reveal the moist, glistening layer beneath. It is suspected—but still unknown—that the treatment stimulates the formation of collagen and elastin, and that production of chemical substances (glycosaminoglycans) plump up the skin's volume. As the exfoliated areas flake and slough off, the result is smoothly resurfaced skin that is firm and glowing.

ARE THERE ANY HEALTH CONSIDERATIONS THAT WOULD DISQUALIFY ME OR INCREASE MY RISK?

If you are pregnant or nursing, check with your doctor, but most recommend against this procedure until pregnancy and/or breast-feeding are completed because the potential for the fetus or baby to absorb the acid is not known. However, because the acid is thought to have no systemic effect, other doctors say it's perfectly safe.

If you are taking Accutane for acne, discontinue the medication at least six months before having a superficial peel.

If you have frequent bouts of the herpes simplex virus (cold sores), you should be prescribed an antiviral agent like Zovirax a few days before the procedure and continue taking it for a week to avoid the blisters that may occur a few days after the application of glycolic acid.

Electrolysis, waxing, and laser hair removal, as well as hair bleaching or the use of depilatories should be discontinued a few days before the procedure.

If you have rosacea or inflamed acne, you run the risk of having the condition worsen because the skin is often too sensitive to withstand chemical exfoliation.

The use of Renova, Retin-A, or similar topical vitamin A products may cause a more exaggerated response to a glycolic acid peel. While some people choose to discontinue using these products a few days before their peel, others are willing to accept the tradeoff of more redness and irritation to achieve a greater degree of skin renewal.

WHO IS A CANDIDATE?

Anyone with mild acne or a tendency toward acne, mild pigment irregularities, superficial fine lines, rough spots, and weather-beaten or sun-damaged skin can benefit from a glycolic acid peel. It can be used on all Fitzpatrick skin types and skin colors (see Chapter 2, "Your Skin, the Sun, and Your Lifestyle").

HOW IS THE PROCEDURE PERFORMED?

All of your makeup is removed and your skin is cleansed with an antiseptic. Then a degreasing agent similar to nail polish remover is applied to eliminate residual oils. You will be given goggles to protect your eyes, and a layer of petroleum jelly is often applied to protect your lips. Then a thin coating of glycolic acid is administered to your face with a gauze pad, swab, or brush. The acid is usually applied from top to bottom: forehead first, followed by cheeks and chin. Often, a fan is used to cool your face and minimize any stinging or burning sensations. An experienced clinician keeps careful track of time and watches for the *first trace* of pinkness, after which the glycolic acid is immediately and *thoroughly* washed off with either tap water or a neutralizing solution that bubbles up and feels quite invigorating. If you feel any areas that are still burning or stinging, additional washing is done. *Note*: Thorough washing is imperative to avoid deeper penetration of the acid and, potentially, increased redness, crusting, and even scarring.

WILL I NEED AN ANESTHETIC?
No. Any mild stinging or burning sensations dissipate in minutes.

HOW LONG DOES THE PROCEDURE TAKE?
About fifteen to thirty minutes.

HOW WILL I LOOK IMMEDIATELY AFTER?
Pink and flushed, like you've run six laps around the track! Sometimes a mild steroid such as hydrocortisone cream is applied to calm down the redness, which may last for a few hours.

HOW WILL I FEEL IMMEDIATELY AFTER?
Refreshed and glowing.

WHAT DOES THE RECOVERY ENTAIL?
Immediately after the peel you can put on moisturizer, sunscreen, and makeup and return to work. Often, a variety of skincare products are prescribed for you to administer at home to enhance the results, for instance hydroquinone to help lighten brown spots, AHA creams to continue gentle exfoliation, and sunscreens to protect against further sun damage. (See Chapter 3, "What's Hot, What's Not, in Skin Care.")

WILL PEOPLE BE ABLE TO TELL THAT I HAVE HAD A PROCEDURE?

Gradually, sun damage will begin to fade and your skin will become more even-toned. You can expect compliments about your healthy glow and clear complexion and questions about the secret of your new radiance.

ARE THERE ANY SIDE EFFECTS, LIMITATIONS, RISKS, OR COMPLICATIONS?

There have been virtually no reported complications or side effects from glycolic acid peels when the acid is applied and removed carefully. If a small amount of glycolic acid inadvertently remains on one area of the skin too long, you may develop crusting or scabbing that can be treated with a topical antibiotic ointment. Pigment changes or scarring are rare.

WHAT DO GLYCOLIC ACID PEELS COST?

Approximately $100 to $150 for each peel, but a package of peels usually brings down the price.

CAN THIS PROCEDURE BE COMBINED WITH OTHER PROCEDURES ON THE SAME DAY?

For deeper, more aggressive peeling, it can be combined with stronger acids such as 25 to 35 percent trichloroacetic acid (TCA) (see Chapter 16, "Not-So-Instant Beauty"), or with microdermabrasion (see Chapter 9, "Rejuvenating Your Skin with a Power Peel"). However, combining a glycolic acid peel with other exfoliating treatments requires a longer recovery period than your typical lunch break allows for.

HOW MANY TREATMENTS WILL I REQUIRE?
A single glycolic acid peel has only minimal effects, which is why people are advised to schedule a series of approximately six peels, administered at weekly or biweekly intervals. After this, many patients sign up for regular maintenance treatments either every other week or once a month to maintain the rejuvenated appearance of their skin.

WHAT CAN I REASONABLY EXPECT?
One or even several *superficial* peels will produce only subtle effects that may be more dramatic to the touch than the eyes. Your skin will feel silky smooth, any freckles and blotchiness will lighten, and acne will improve. However, if you want wrinkle relief and real drama, you may want to consider a deeper chemical peel, dermabrasion, or a laser peel. (See Chapter 16, "Not-So-Instant Beauty.")

ARE THERE ALTERNATIVES TO GLYCOLIC ACID PEELS WITH SIMILAR RESULTS?
Applying dry ice–like liquid nitrogen or carbon dioxide slush can superficially freeze the top layer of the skin, causing it to slough off. Microdermabrasion is a mechanical method of super-ficially sanding and buffing the skin to achieve similar results. (See Chapter 9, "Rejuvenating Your Skin with a Power Peel.")

Salicylic acid, also known as beta hydroxy acid (BHA), is found naturally in willow bark, sweet birch bark, and winter-green leaves, and has been used safely for decades as a peeling agent. Unlike AHAs that are water-soluble, BHAs are fat-soluble, making them extremely effective in the treatment of acne, among other conditions.

TCA (10 to 20 percent). Anything stronger is not considered a superficial peel but rather a medium or deep peel because redness can last for days before the skin crusts and peels. (See Chapter 16, "Not-So-Instant Beauty.")

Jessner's solution—a combination of resorcinol, salicylic acid, and lactic acid in an alcohol solution—is a lunchtime procedure when applied lightly. If the solution is applied heavily, there is greater depth of penetration into the skin and so greater exfoliation, but recovery takes about a week. The number of coats applied is determined by the patient's work schedule and desire for rapid results. A series of treatments can soften fine lines, eliminate blackheads, and improve hyperpigmentation such as the "mask of pregnancy."

If you listen to your psychic the way Danielle did, you, too, may postpone a glycolic acid peel for a month in order to concentrate less on yourself than on other matters. To her, it was worth the wait. When she finally went back to her soothsayer, the woman predicted great things. "I see a glowing future," she said.

rejuvenating your skin with a power peel

the power peel and other microdermabrasion techniques that give your skin polish and pizzazz

You've been there or you've heard about them, those power lunches where big-time movers and shakers thrust and parry, wheel and deal, make daring decisions and change the world. But most significant changes—in your personal or professional life—often take time: sometimes months, sometimes years.

Not so the skin power peel, which can be accomplished during a single lunch break. If you're a wheeler and dealer, wanting to make and also to look like a million dollars, but you don't have the time to indulge in months of rejuvenating cosmetic therapy, the power peel may be just what you're looking for.

It certainly did the trick for Justine, a former college track star and mother of four. The high-powered state assemblywoman had always enjoyed vibrant health and what seemed like ageless beauty.

"Everyone, and I mean everyone, used to tell me how young I looked, and they'd marvel when they learned that my kids were out of college and I was even a grandmother," she said. "But one of my neighbors told me that I'd know when that dewy look was gone. I had no idea what she was talking about until this year, when I hit fifty. Now I know, and I hate it."

In truth, the change in Justine wasn't dramatic. Except for some subtle crow's feet and fine lines and only the slightest sagging of her enviable jawline, she still looked as amazing in her skin-tight gym outfit as she did in a slinky cocktail dress. Nevertheless, the compliments had abated, and Justine, who looked at her face in a triple magnification mirror every morning, knew why.

"It was the whole look of my skin," she said. "It looked dull and sallow; it had tiny rough spots and brown blotches. My pores were clogged, and a scar that always bothered me was looking worse. I just didn't have what everyone used to call my old pizzazz."

Always solution-oriented, Justine was determined to recapture her old sparkle. She tried over-the-counter moisturizers containing retinol to bring the glow back to her skin. She bought Buf-Pufs and other exfoliating agents to get rid of her rough spots. And she used Bioré strips to clean out her pores. The net result was a minor improvement, but she still hated the way her skin looked.

One day Justine bumped into a legislative colleague in the state capitol, a woman of forty-seven, and was struck by her radiant complexion. "You look incredible!" she told her colleague, blurting out the problems she was having with her own skin. "What's your secret?"

"If microdermabrasion was once a secret," the woman answered, "it isn't anymore. I've been telling so many people about it that I should be getting an agent's fee from my dermatologist!"

The woman told Justine that she had suffered from adult acne and was constantly annoyed by the tiny pink and red bumps on her face. "I felt like I was revisiting my adolescence," she said, grimacing at the memory. "Even when the pimples went away, my skin looked stained, and the tone of my complexion looked completely uneven."

The microdermabrasion Justine's dermatologist recommended turned out to be the satisfying solution she had been looking for. After only six lunchtime sessions, her "buffed" skin looked as youthful as her buff body, and she, too, became a walking advertisement for the procedure.

questions and answers about microdermabrasion

WHAT IS MICRODERMABRASION?
Microdermabrasion—also known as skin buffing, polishing, sandblasting, or particle-beam resurfacing—is a mechanical method of bombarding the most superficial layer of skin (the stratum corneum) with a spray of aluminum oxide crystals (also known as corundum). After the skin on the face, hands, neck, or décolleté is exfoliated and sloughs off, it is replaced by a new layer of rejuvenated skin. Several companies manufacture microdermabrasion machines, and the procedure is commonly described by their seductive names: Power Peel, Gentle Peel, SmartPeel, MegaPeel, Parisian Peel, UltraPeel, DermaPeel—the list goes on. While the European market has been using microdermabrasion since the late 1980s, it was introduced in the United States only in 1997.

WHO IS A CANDIDATE?
Anyone who wants to improve the appearance of his or her skin, even up irregular skin tones, or restore luster to dull, lifeless skin is a candidate. Since the stratum corneum layer of skin on the face is constantly exposed to environmental stressors like wind, cold,

sun, smoke, and pollution, it is not necessary to have a clinical "condition" to avail yourself of microdermabrasion's cosmetically enhancing effects. The procedure is particularly helpful for those with mild acne or acne-prone skin, blackheads, brown blotches from sun damage, and the facial "mask of pregnancy." It is sometimes helpful in improving the appearance of wrinkles, scars, stretch marks, and enlarged pores.

ARE THERE ANY DISQUALIFYING CONSIDERATIONS?

Anyone who is taking Accutane should not have microdermabrasion until the medication has been discontinued for six months. Otherwise, it is a safe procedure for most skin types, including types IV and V. (See Fitzpatrick scale in Chapter 2, "Your Skin, the Sun, and Your Lifestyle.")

ARE THERE ALTERNATIVES TO MICRODERMABRASION?

Chemical exfoliation that uses a mild acid to peel the top layers of the skin can bring about a similar effect (see Chapter 8, "Feeling Refreshed with Chemical Peels"). Those who administer chemical peels, however, usually don't have the same kind of control over the areas that are treated as those who administer microdermabrasion, which is performed mechanically, thereby allowing the clinician to concentrate with great precision on specific, discrete areas. Numerous over-the-counter topical scrubs containing abrasive ingredients like apricot pits, salt, sugar, or even tiny diamond particles can also gently exfoliate the top layers of the skin. Some of these products may also contain active ingredients like alpha or beta hydroxy acids that can bring about further exfoliation. Some doctors use fine sandpaper to achieve similar results. But this is nothing new. Ancient Egyptians used sandpaper to abrade scars in 1500 B.C..

HOW DO I PREPARE FOR MICRODERMABRASION?

About two or three days before the procedure, stop using Retin-A, Renova, or any product that contains glycolic acid or a topical exfoliating scrub, all of which increase the skin's fragility and may also increase the irritation and redness that follow the microdermabrasion procedure.

WHAT IS THE BEST TIME TO HAVE MICRODERMABRASION?

Lunchtime, of course! It's a short procedure with immediately visible results. But if you are planning a special occasion, schedule the treatment a few days ahead of time in case your skin gets mildly ruddy immediately after the procedure.

HOW IS THE PROCEDURE PERFORMED?

Microdermabrasion (*micro* = "tiny [crystals]," *derm* = "skin," *abrasion* = "scraping") is performed with a specialized machine that mixes small particles of aluminum oxide crystals and sprays them out of a sterilized handpiece onto all areas of the face. After the skin has been gently exfoliated, the crystals and dead skin cells are suctioned back into a closed receptacle through a vacuumlike device. The practitioner may customize each treatment by regulating the flow of crystals and the power of the vacuum. In addition to cleansing the face, pulling out blackheads, and unclogging pores, the treatment stimulates blood flow, lymphatic circulation, and the growth of new skin cells and collagen.

WILL I NEED AN ANESTHETIC?

No. However, when the crystals first make contact with your face, you may experience a mild but very tolerable scratchy sensation, and after the procedure you may feel the same kind of tingling or stinging that comes from mild sunburn.

HOW DOES MICRODERMABRASION DIFFER FROM DERMABRASION?

They are like apples and oranges. Microdermabrasion, a bloodless procedure performed with a spray of aluminum oxide crystals, is a method of *superficial* exfoliation that is not associated with any downtime. Dermabrasion, performed with a rapidly rotating wheel studded with tiny diamond particles, abrades the skin much more deeply, causing bleeding, oozing, and crusting of the skin. Recovery from dermabrasion takes at least two weeks (see Chapter 16, "Not-So-Instant Beauty"). The final results of the two procedures are also like night and day. The clinical effects of microdermabrasion are subtle, whereas the improvement in wrinkles and acne scars after dermabrasion can be quite dramatic.

CAN MICRODERMABRASION BE COMBINED WITH OTHER PROCEDURES DURING THE SAME SESSION?

The treatment is sometimes performed immediately before a glycolic acid peel to achieve greater improvement in the appearance of fine lines and blotchy pigmentation, but side effects like a burning sensation or possible crusting of the skin may occur and downtime may involve a few days and not the minutes or hours of simple microdermabrasion alone. Microdermabrasion can also be combined with nonablative laser treatments like the CoolTouch, or N-Lite. (See Chapter 12, "Nonablative Lasers for Wrinkles.") In essence, you're targeting the epidermis with microdermabrasion, and the dermis with nonablative laser treatment for maximal skin rejuvenation.

WHAT SPECIAL TRAINING IS REQUIRED?

The regulations of each state determine who can use microdermabrasion machines. Licensed aestheticians and registered nurses who have special training in the technique commonly perform the procedure, using machines that are preset to abrade only the most superficial layer of skin. However, only board-certified dermatologists, plastic surgeons, and physicians with in-depth knowledge of the skin are qualified to use the turbo settings of the machine to perform a more aggressive treatment that penetrates the skin's deeper layers. But with deeper peels, there is usually some bleeding and crusting of the skin and a longer recovery period than is typical of the lunchtime procedure. It cannot be overstated that the qualifications of the person who administers your treatment are extremely important because there is a small but real potential risk for scarring if a poorly trained or unskilled clinician uses too much suction or is too aggressive in administering the aluminum oxide crystals. (See Chapter 4, "Better Safe Than Sorry.")

HOW WILL I LOOK IMMEDIATELY AFTER?

Your skin may be reddish or pinkish for anywhere from about thirty minutes to a full day, and there may be a temporary streaking of redness and mild swelling, depending on the extent of the procedure. Occasionally, there may be a tiny bruise if the suction vacuum inadvertently pinches the skin. Many skin-care products, such as moisturizers containing antioxidants, are beneficial after microdermabrasion because they penetrate the skin more effectively than they did when the skin's dead cells created a barrier to absorption. (See Chapter 3, "What's Hot, What's Not, in Skin Care.")

HOW WILL I FEEL IMMEDIATELY AFTER?
Both you and your skin will feel tingly, rejuvenated, relaxed, cleansed, and invigorated.

HOW LONG DOES THE PROCEDURE TAKE?
From start to finish, each treatment lasts approximately twenty to thirty minutes.

HOW MANY TREATMENTS WILL I REQUIRE?
For optimal results and to maintain the thrill of polished glistening skin and a glowing youthful look, a series of six to ten treatments is often recommended, administered weekly or biweekly, and maintenance sessions are often performed throughout the year.

WHAT DOES THE RECOVERY ENTAIL?
There is no recovery period. Immediately after the procedure, you can apply moisturizers, sunscreen, and makeup and go back to your life!

WILL PEOPLE BE ABLE TO TELL THAT I HAVE HAD A PROCEDURE DONE?
Don't be surprised if your friends, coworkers, and loved ones remark on how terrific you look, how smooth and unlined your skin appears, that your pores seem smaller, and that you have a beautiful glow. But the beauty and subtlety of microdermabrasion are that people are more apt to think that you've gone on a relaxing vacation than had a cosmetic procedure. When you—or they—touch your skin, it will feel as smooth as velvet.

DOES MICRODERMABRASION LEAVE SCARS?
When performed carefully and correctly, the answer is no. In fact, a series of treatments often improves scars and stretch marks.

HOW LONG WILL THE RESULTS LAST?
About one or two weeks.

WHAT ARE THE LIMITATIONS, RISKS, OR COMPLICATIONS?
The procedure is noninvasive and considered extremely safe if performed by qualified professionals.

ARE THERE ANY SPECIAL CONCERNS FOR WOMEN OF COLOR?
Treatment that is too aggressive or that invades the skin too deeply has the potential to cause hyperpigmentation, especially if the skin is exposed to the sun.

ARE THE CRYSTALS THAT ARE USED IN MICRODERMABRASION SAFE?
The easy answer is yes, but it bears elaboration. Ever since the method made its debut in the United States in the late 1990s, overzealous and alarmist journalists have erroneously linked aluminum oxide crystals to Alzheimer's disease, basing their reports largely on studies dating back to 1965 that have since been discredited by the advent of electron microscopes that are now able to chart the chemistry and genetics of brain conditions with amazing precision. In spite of dozens of articles in scientific, peer-reviewed journals that have refuted the Alzheimer's-aluminum link, and in spite of the fact that the FDA has never

even discussed taking aluminum oxide off the market, there continues to be a flood of advertising touting the use of "safe alternatives."

And here is the ultimate irony: Aluminum oxide contains no aluminum! It is categorized as a ceramic that is commonly found in everything from antacids to antiperspirants, buffered aspirin to lipsticks, canned foods to toothpaste, canned soda to vegetable oils, and even tap water. It is also used in orthopedic implants, dental implants, and tooth abrasion. In fact, for more than fifty years, dentists have been safely shooting aluminum oxide crystals directly into the mouths of their patients with no adverse health effects. Still, manufacturers of "alternatives" continue to offer a variety of "gentler" abrasive materials such as sodium bicarbonate (baking soda), sodium chloride (table salt), and magnesium oxide (found in sea water). Several companies have developed new microdermabrasion machines that eliminate the sprays of aluminum oxide and other particles onto the skin. Instead, diamond-encrusted wands are used to vacuum the skin, resulting in the benefits of abrasion without the gritty residue left by the aluminum oxide particles.

WHAT DOES MICRODERMABRASION COST?

The cost in a salon or spa is about $175 to $200 per treatment. In a doctor's office, it is usually about $250 per session, but a "package" of multiple treatments may bring down the fee. Do-it-yourselfers should be aware of the Dermanew microdermabrasion system, the first handheld system that can be used at home.

WHAT CAN I REASONABLY EXPECT?

If you trust many of the computer-enhanced, hyped-up before-and-after photographs that *seem* to demonstrate dramatic— indeed, miraculous—improvements of wrinkles or acne scars, you will be disappointed with microdermabrasion, because only deeper chemical peels or carbon dioxide laser resurfacing can achieve these results. (See Chapter 16, "Not-So-Instant Beauty.") But you can realistically expect a visible improvement of adult acne, greatly enhanced skin texture, a fresher appearance, the feeling that your face is exquisitely clean, and lots of compliments.

Ironically, patients love the procedure more than doctors do. Many physicians say that it is difficult for them to actually see much improvement. Accustomed as they are to bringing about dramatic changes, they feel that microdermabrasion lies more in the realm of the emperor's new clothes than in any empirical results. But don't tell that to patients who swear by the procedure!

banishing cellulite

the real "skinny" about Endermologie and
other methods of treating cellulite

Some people have the no-fat diet down to a science. Having memorized, and avoided, all the foods that contain those ever-threatening fat grams, they buy dairy fat substitutes, create wonderful dishes that look and, they say, taste mouth-wateringly delicious, and eat plenty of fill-the-stomach salads and vegetables with, of course, no-fat dressing. And to augment their aversion to fat, they exercise daily and thrill at the image of any residual body fat dripping off their frames as they sweat it out.

Janie, a forty-year-old health maven, is such a person, a woman you would think everyone would envy. With big brains, big breasts, a svelte figure, professional success as a Wall Street broker, a loving husband, two great kids, and a sparkling personality, she could have been downright intimidating. But she wasn't, largely because her Corn Belt upbringing had endowed her with both a down-to-earth quality and modesty about her formidable accomplishments.

"I owe it all to my thighs!" she would say. And everyone would laugh and say, "Right!" When they looked at Janie, in all of her shapely, earthy, size-twelve glory, they appreciated her self-deprecating humor but they didn't believe it for a minute.

But Janie knew better. She hadn't worn a bathing suit since her honeymoon. Although her work and home life kept her too busy to obsess about the dimpled, rippled, cellulite-ridden bane of her life, she detested her thighs. The regular exercises she did on her walking machine hadn't helped, and when she was thirty-nine, she started to look at her thighs in a new—and even more horrified—way.

"It was an out-of-body experience," she said. "I didn't know who these things belonged to—certainly not me!" Late one evening, she accessed her favorite search engine on the Internet and typed in "thighs." In seconds, the word *Endermologie* popped up. Janie was riveted.

She learned that in the late 1970s, a French inventor named Louis Paul Guitay suffered muscle and skin damage in a car accident, and the scarring that resulted was treated by therapeutic massage to soften his tissues and scars and restore muscle function and elasticity. His massage sessions lasted from three to four hours a day and involved a rigorous routine of manually rolling the skin. Dissatisfied with these time-consuming and labor-intensive treatments and with the fact that his progress seemed to depend on the skill of a particular therapist, Guitay designed the Endermologie system, which was first manufactured by the LPG company in France.

The mechanical method of massage proved to be more effective than manual massage, and it was not long before doctors in Europe, Japan, South America, and the United States began treating trauma and burn patients with Guitay's noninvasive, nonsurgical Endermologie machines and noticing incidentally that the treatment seemed to reduce the appearance of cellulite and alter fat distribution. They didn't understand the phenomenon, but they theorized that the technique's extreme pressure and rolling motion damaged subcutaneous fat cells and that the healing process resulted in an improved contour of the skin and better distribution of subcutaneous fat. They also noticed that only the fat layer was altered, and not the overlying skin or underlying bones and muscles.

"I figured if horrible thighs are what God gave me," Janie said, "it was wrong to be ungrateful for all my blessings by complaining that a relatively small physical defect meant that much."

Yet in spite of her evolved philosophy, Endermologie proved irresistible, especially when she learned that the device was first marketed in the United States in 1996, after approval by the FDA. The following week, Janie met with an aesthetician in the office of a Manhattan dermatologist. Questions in hand, many of them gleaned from her Internet browsing, she wanted to know what she would have to invest in Endermologie and what its potential risks and expected returns were.

questions and answers about Endermologie

WHAT IS ENDERMOLOGIE?
It is a technique of mechanical massage that reduces the appearance of cellulite. While technology that is similar to Guitay's performs the same function, the word *Endermologie* has become popularly associated with the treatment, much like Kleenex and Xerox have become almost generic terms for tissues and photocopying.

WHAT EXACTLY IS CELLULITE?
Cellulite, a term coined in European salons and spas to describe deposits of dimpled fat found on the thighs and buttocks of many women, has never been precisely or even adequately defined in

medical literature. It is not a medical term, and many doctors don't acknowledge that such a condition exists but attribute it to ordinary deposits of fatty tissue. On the other hand, spa and salon owners claim that cellulite is "fat gone wrong" that involves a combination of fat, water, and toxic wastes that the body has failed to eliminate.

Most physicians, however, do acknowledge that cellulite is a "woman's thing," that females are anatomically different from men in significant ways, and that even skinny women are vulnerable to developing lumpy, bumpy thighs and buttocks. In fact, more than 90 percent of women after puberty are plagued by the *peau d'orange* (orange peel), quilted, lumpy, bumpy contour of their thighs, hips, and buttocks.

Doctors believe that strands of fibrous tissue anchor the skin to deeper tissue layers and that they also divide the fat cells into compartments. When fat cells increase in size, these compartments bulge and produce a waffled appearance of the skin.

Many practitioners of Endermologie believe that the deep massage technique pulls water out of the fatty tissues and back into normal circulation, increases blood flow in the skin that stimulates enzymes to break down the trapped fat cells, speeds up the body's metabolism to burn fat in the areas of treatment, and increases lymphatic drainage to help the body eliminate the by-products of fat metabolism.

WHO IS A CANDIDATE?

Any woman of normal weight or, at most, twenty pounds overweight. If you are more than twenty pounds overweight, the ripples of cellulite may be dealt with more effectively by dieting. Generally, Endermologie works best for women under age forty-five. It is especially helpful after liposuction in restoring improved contour to the thighs and buttocks. (See Chapter 16, "Not-So-Instant Beauty.")

WHAT HEALTH CONSIDERATIONS OR RISKS WOULD DISQUALIFY ME?

Endermologie is not recommended for anyone taking a blood-thinning medication like Coumadin or who has a bleeding disorder or bruises easily. Pregnant women should not have the procedure because its effect on the developing fetus is unknown, but the massage technique helps after delivery in getting back into shape and improving skin tone.

HOW DO I PREPARE FOR ENDERMOLOGIE?

The only preparation is to find a qualified "endermologist" who has experience in the technique. These may include physicians, licensed aestheticians, registered nurses, personal trainers, and ancillary medical personnel who have been trained in the technique. The manufacturer of the Endermologie machine sponsors courses and awards certificates to those who complete the training. But be aware that Endermologie, like many cosmetic treatments, requires a certain degree of artistry. In other words, successful Endermologie is technique dependent. Make sure that the practitioner you choose has been fully trained.

WHAT DOES AN ENDERMOLOGIE TREATMENT ENTAIL?

You lie on a treatment table, either on your stomach or back, and the therapist applies the handheld Endermologie machine to the areas of cellulite. The machine consists of two motorized rollers and a powerful suction hose that draw up, fold, and knead the tissues. The vacuum hose glides over the skin, creating a warm ironing effect or a feeling of deep massage while it increases circulation, improves skin tone, and reduces the appearance of cellulite. The machine's settings range from mild to intensive, allowing the practitioner to vary the treatment to your comfort level. Before the treatment, you are given special stretch panty hose to put on, over which the machine can glide smoothly. Occasionally, some sensitivity in the front of the thighs is experienced, but nothing that would require even an aspirin. Photographs are taken both before and after treatment to provide an accurate record of improvements.

WILL I NEED AN ANESTHETIC?
No. The treatment is not associated with any pain.

HOW LONG WILL THE PROCEDURE TAKE?
A typical treatment lasts thirty-five minutes.

HOW MANY TREATMENTS WILL I REQUIRE?
The Endermologie machine's manufacturer recommends about twenty treatments, starting with twice-a-week appointments that are followed by biweekly or monthly maintenance sessions. In April 2000, the FDA allowed the LPG company to state that the treatment can "temporarily" improve the appearance of cellulite and reduce the circumference of cellulite-treated areas. This is because the effects will dissipate and cellulite will reappear in anyone who discontinues the treatment for a month or two.

HOW WILL I LOOK IMMEDIATELY AFTER?
Any treated area may be slightly reddened. If the Endermologie machine has been turned to a higher setting, you may see some bruising from small broken blood vessels, which will disappear in a few days. If you are planning to wear a bikini, short shorts, or a micro-mini skirt, it's better to plan your treatment a few days ahead. Topical vitamin K cream can speed the healing process.

HOW WILL I FEEL IMMEDIATELY AFTER?
Invigorated, revitalized, and relaxed.

CAN ENDERMOLOGIE BE COMBINED WITH OTHER PROCEDURES?
After liposuction, a series of twenty Endermologie treatments often improves the appearance of cellulite and hastens the reduction of swelling. Liposuction is an invasive procedure that vacuums out excess fat through a cannula that is inserted into small incisions, but it is not a cure for cellulite. While liposuction may decrease the circumference of the thighs, in some people it may worsen the texture of the skin and make cellulite more visible. Endermologie treatments often shorten the recovery period after liposuction. (See Chapter 16, "Not-So-Instant Beauty.")

WHAT CAN I REASONABLY EXPECT FROM ENDERMOLOGIE TREATMENTS?
After about six to eight sessions—depending on the individual—there may be a range of results, from subtle cellulite reduction and better skin tone to a dramatic reduction in the girth of the thighs; a slimmer, trimmer figure; and even a smaller dress or pants size. You will see less dimpling, puckering, loose skin, and cottage cheese areas. And many patients say that losing weight is easier because the treatments motivate them to follow a moderate exercise regimen, eat a more sensible low-fat diet, and drink eight—yes, eight!—glasses of water every day, which fill the stomach and reduce the appetite.

Another motivating factor is that each time an Endermologie treatment is administered, the patient is weighed and her body measurements taken. While clinicians don't know why Endermologie works so well for so many people, it's safe to say that the treatments along with diet, exercise, and water drinking are a magical combination.

ARE THERE ALTERNATIVES TO
ENDERMOLOGIE TREATMENTS?

A variety of creams and herbs promise to reduce cellulite, but none have been subject to double-blind crossover studies or approved by the FDA. Some creams contain caffeine or similar agents that have a diuretic effect, drawing water from the skin that creates a temporary reduction in the appearance of cellulite, but they have not shown any long-term effects. Many creams are simply moisturizers or exfoliators containing retinol or AHAs that may temporarily firm up the skin but have no effect on the underlying fat.

Many spas offer body wraps that promise an instant melting away of fat and an immediate loss of weight and inches, but the weight loss is actually temporary water loss from perspiration.

Electric muscle stimulators (EMS) are medical devices, approved by the FDA for relaxing muscle spasms, increasing blood circulation, and rehabilitating muscle function after a stroke. Many spas and salons claim that EMS can remove wrinkles, increase bust size, and remove cellulite through electric shocks that are delivered to the muscles. However, the FDA considers promotion of muscle stimulators for any type of body shaping, contouring, or spot reducing to be fraudulent.

Cellasene, an anticellulite pill that arrived in U.S. pharmacies in 1999, features ingredients like ginkgo biloba, sweet clover, grape seed extract, bioflavinoids, evening primrose oil, fish oil, soya oil, and bladder wrack (a form of seaweed) that may have diuretic effects. But only three studies about the efficacy of the pill have been conducted involving a total of one hundred women. The manufacturer of the pill sponsored the studies, but none have been published in peer-reviewed medical journals. Many experienced dermatologists are loathe to recommend Cellasene to their patients because some of its ingredients have powerful anticlotting properties that are potentially dangerous if taken with aspirin or blood thinners. And one ingredient, bladder wrack, contains significant amounts of iodine that could adversely affect the thyroid gland, cause a flare-up of acne, and be dangerous to those allergic to it.

The latest fad to come along is CelluLite Fashion Hosiery. The company claims that the panty hose it manufactures features an ingredient that metabolizes fatty tissues. The hosiery must be worn all day for eight weeks to reap the full benefit. Long-term, double-blind studies have yet to be done. Remember, the cheapest and most effective cellulite buster is still a healthy diet and aerobic activity.

WILL PEOPLE BE ABLE TO TELL THAT I HAVE HAD ENDERMOLOGIE TREATMENTS?

Unless the combination of Endermologie treatments and a comprehensive weight loss and exercise program transforms you from a size sixteen to a size twelve, it is unlikely that people will notice a difference in the way you look in clothing. But *you* will notice the changes in how your slacks fit and feel more confident when you wear shorts or a bathing suit. Studies as to the efficacy of the treatments are mixed, with some reporting significant reduction in body circumference and others reporting none.

HOW LONG WILL THE RESULTS LAST?

If you continue the Endermologie treatments on a monthly or a twice-monthly maintenance program, the results will last indefinitely. But if you discontinue the treatments, your original skin tone and cellulite will return.

WHAT DO ENDERMOLOGIE TREATMENTS COST?

In a doctor's office, each treatment costs approximately $100, but there is usually a discount if you buy a package of approximately twenty treatments.

WHAT IS THE SATISFACTION RATE FROM ENDERMOLOGIE TREATMENTS?

It is high for those who are ideal candidates to begin with and who stick with the program and have realistic expectations. The most satisfied customers diet and exercise to lose weight at the same time that they're having their treatments.

IS THERE ANYTHING ELSE I SHOULD KNOW ABOUT ENDERMOLOGIE?

Don't be fooled by advertisements that tout a "new, cellulite-free you" with Endermologie treatments alone. When the LPG company produced its first brochure featuring dramatic photographs of cellulite-ridden people before they had undergone Endermologie and impressive photographs of their shapely bodies after treatment, the public believed that these painless treatments were the answer to their dreams. The media responded immediately with uncritical abandon, touting the new technology and creating a virtual craze based more on hype than reality.

The reality turned out to be that the company had omitted the fact that in addition to twenty Endermologie treatments, the people in the photographs had had liposuction and significant weight loss over a period of several months. Ultimately, the FDA mandated that the company pull its brochures off the market and correct its misleading information.

The lesson is clear: The amount of fat in the body is determined by an individual's eating and exercise habits, but the distribution of fat is determined by hormones and heredity. People with cellulite can, indeed, have successful Endermologie treatments, but not without embracing auxiliary lifestyle changes.

part three

the miracle of lasers

laser treatment of brown blemishes

also age spots, birthmarks,
and tattoos

Everyone who has ever sat down to a meal or enjoyed a midnight snack can attest to the tastiness of leftovers. The same cannot be said, however, about the leftover signs of aging and damage that the sun leaves on the faces of just about every man and woman on the planet. Sunspots (also called age or liver spots) mar the appearance and make people look older than they are. The good news is that it takes only a few minutes to get rid of them.

Maddy finally did. She had gone through the first fifty years of her life being called all the *m* words: marvelous, miracle woman, magnanimous, maven, and Mother Earth—and for good reason. Married at nineteen to George, a retailer of men's clothing, they had raised two children of their own and four physically handicapped children they had adopted.

To make ends meet, Maddy made many of the clothes her children wore and planted her own version of the victory garden her mother had planted during World War II. It helped that the family lived in sunny Florida where they could plant year-round.

And it was a perfect pursuit for the whole family, with some of the children driving stakes for tomato plants, green beans, and corn, others aligning strings to make sure the carrots and radishes came up in straight rows, still others spreading fertilizer or picking insects off the leaves every evening.

When she finally came in from her days in the sun, Maddy baked delectable loaves of zucchini bread and filled jars of tomato sauce that she sold to local gourmet shops and also served to her family or put in her freezer for future use. She and her family flourished and, of course, always looked the picture of suntanned health. While they didn't have much money for expensive diversions, they often spent evenings playing board games and charades.

By the time Maddy was forty-eight, her children were grown and employed in jobs that included lawyer, supermarket checker, registered nurse, rehabilitation therapist, gas station attendant, and sous chef. One Easter, when they were all together, her oldest daughter suggested that they play a new game: What Animal Do I Look Like?

"I'll start," the young woman said. "I already know that I look like a rabbit!" Everyone laughed. Then one of Maddy's sons piped up, "Mom is easy—she looks like a leopard!"

"Perfect!" Maddy chortled, dubbing herself with two more *m* words. "I'll even call myself the mottled missus." It was true. The years in the sun, unprotected by sunscreen, had left Maddy's face, hands, neck, and cleavage covered with brown spots.

"Mom," her registered nurse daughter chimed in, "you can get rid of those and look a whole lot younger at the same time." She told her about "the miracle" of laser surgery and that, even if she didn't have it, she should have her spots checked out to be sure they weren't skin cancer.

It didn't take much convincing. Within a week, Maddy was at the dermatologist's office, very relieved that none of her spots were cancer and very curious about being spot-free and looking younger.

questions and answers about pigment-specific laser treatments

WHAT ARE AGE SPOTS?

They are light or dark brown spots on the tops of the hands, face, shoulders, chin, upper chest, and any other areas that are or have been chronically exposed to the sun. As we age, chronic sun exposure alters the function of the cells in the skin. The melanocytes (*melano* = "color," *cyte* = "cell") that arise from the basal layer of the epidermis produce the color-bearing pigment called melanin. As the production of melanin becomes irregular and sporadic, pigment clumps together, causing brown spots that give the skin a mottled or blotchy appearance. To appreciate the harmful effects of the sun, simply compare the smooth, unblemished skin on the breasts and buttocks or other areas of the body that are always covered by clothing to the irregularly pigmented skin in sun-exposed areas. Even if a woman has had a facelift that makes her appear years younger than her chronological age, her hands will be a dead giveaway in revealing her true age. Happily, pigment-specific lasers can reverse years—even decades— of sun damage.

WHO IS A CANDIDATE FOR TREATMENT WITH THE PIGMENT-SPECIFIC LASER?

Anyone with age spots—sort of. Why this disclaimer? Because it's a complete waste of time and money to undergo laser treatment for age spots if there is not a commitment to stay out of the sun and off tanning beds forever! With subsequent exposure to the sun, age spots will recur and new ones will develop.

ARE THERE ALTERNATIVES TO THE PROCEDURE?

- Topical Retin-A or Renova.
- Hydroquinone and other bleaching agents.
- Alpha hydroxy acids and other exfoliating agents.
- Electrodesiccation and curettage that destroys pigment cells with a mild electric current and then scrapes them away. However, the process may damage normal surrounding skin and result in textural or pigment changes and scarring if the electrocautery machine's current is too high or remains on the skin for too long.
- Liquid nitrogen (cryosurgery) freezes age spots, but if applied too lightly they remain and if applied overzealously permanent loss of pigmentation can give the skin a white, scarlike appearance.
- Trichloracetic acid (TCA) and other acids peel away the top layers of skin.

While any of these treatments can be used to treat age spots, the pigment-specific lasers are by far the most effective.

HOW DO I PREPARE FOR MY PROCEDURE?

The best preparation is to swear off sun exposure forever. In addition to applying sunscreen to the face, it is important to coat the tops of the hands and the exposed area of the chest every day.

HOW IS THE PROCEDURE PERFORMED?

The beam of light from a pigment-specific laser (such as the Q-switched ruby, the Q-switched alexandrite, or the Q-switched Nd:YAG) is targeted at each brown spot. The specific pigment in the spot acts as a magnet, drawing the light only to the pigment while sparing the surrounding skin any damage.

WILL I NEED AN ANESTHETIC?

If a large number of age spots on the hand, arms, legs, chest, or face are being treated at one session, EMLA cream or injections of local anesthesia can numb the area. The sensation of the laser is often compared to the snapping of a rubber band on the skin— tolerable at best, briefly irritating at worst.

HOW WILL I LOOK IMMEDIATELY AFTER?

During treatment a tiny amount of pinpoint bleeding may occur as well as minimal local swelling. Immediately after treatment, each site becomes reddish and begins to form a scab. By the next day, once the scab has fully formed, you can apply coverup makeup to camouflage the treated sites.

HOW LONG DOES THE PROCEDURE TAKE?

A few to thirty minutes, depending on the number of age spots. Since the laser fires rapidly, numerous age spots can be treated quickly and efficiently. After a single treatment those dead give-aways of age are gone and your face and/or hands will appear many years younger as literally years of sun damage vanish in minutes.

HOW MANY TREATMENTS WILL I REQUIRE?

Usually one, but if a few spots have to be touched up, another session may be needed.

WHAT DOES THE RECOVERY ENTAIL?

Immediately after treatment, ice packs can soothe the sites that were lased. Antibiotic ointment is applied in small amounts to the crusted sites and care is taken not to scrub the skin. Sometimes a bandage or dressing is placed over the sites to help protect the area. The difference in healing times depends on the blood supply to each area: age spots on the face take about a week to heal; on the arms and chest, about two weeks; and on the lower extremities or tops of the hands about three weeks. As the tiny scabs fall off, the skin appears light pink in some of the treated areas and it may take a month or two for this discoloration to disappear completely. It is imperative to continue to use sunscreen and avoid direct sun exposure for several months after treatment. If you're thinking about having all of your age spots removed before summertime when your skin will be on display, give yourself a couple of months lead time.

HOW LONG WILL THE RESULTS LAST?
With strict sun precautions, potentially forever.

ARE THERE ANY LIMITATIONS, SIDE EFFECTS, OR RISKS?
Overwhelmingly, age spots are exactly what they appear to be. But sometimes, they're not. If the diagnosis of your skin problem is unclear or what doctors call "suspicious," your dermatologist will recommend a biopsy to rule out the possibility of malignant melanoma. If you have an olive or darker complexion, hyperpigmentation (or a temporary darkening of the skin) may occur after treatment, but that doesn't mean the treatment has failed. Patience, avoidance of the sun, and bleaching cream will help. In a couple of months the darkening will vanish and you will see that the laser has eliminated your sunspots. Transient hypopigmentation (or lightening of the skin) is less common, but it can occur. Camouflage makeup is helpful until your natural pigment returns.

WHAT DOES THE PROCEDURE COST?

Cost ranges from a few hundred dollars on up, depending on the number of age spots treated, the number of pulses emitted by the laser, and the time involved in the treatment.

ARE THERE OTHER CONDITIONS AMENABLE TO TREATMENT WITH PIGMENT-SPECIFIC LASERS?

Café-au-lait spots are flat, light brown or tan lesions (the color, aptly, of coffee with milk) that are always benign but a cosmetic nuisance. About 10 percent of children are born with one or more café-au-lait spots or develop them in childhood. However, in the rare case that a baby is born with more than six café-au-lait spots, he or she must be evaluated to rule out the uncommon but devastating condition of neurofibromatosis. In addition, because melanocytes in the skin develop from neural origins, the appearance of a large number of these spots may mean the patient will develop numerous neurofibromas and other neurological symptoms. If a patient has a café-au-lait spot that is cosmetically disturbing, treatment with a pigment-specific laser is often helpful. The treatment is quick and easy, requiring from two to ten sessions spaced from four to eight weeks apart. The goal of the treatment is to destroy all of the pigment in order to decrease the rate of recurrence. However, even after several laser treatments, the cure rate is only about 50 percent because café-au-lait spots have a tendency to recur within several weeks to several months in the same shape and distribution as the original lesions.

Becker's nevi are flat light brown cosmetically disfiguring discolorations found in 0.5 percent of the population. They usually develop during puberty and adolescence, typically on the torso and shoulders of teenagers. Although similar in appearance to café-au-lait spots, they are significantly larger, covering an extensive area of the body. Treatment with a pigment-specific laser may be effective in lightening or removing nevi, but they have a high rate of recurrence.

Postinflammatory hyperpigmentation may occur following any type of trauma. For instance, a fall from a bike may result in a scab developing on a scraped knee or leg. Once healed, a brown stain may persist for many months or longer. Similar staining can occur on the face after a rash or an outbreak of acne has gone away. People with olive complexions often experience severe postinflammatory hyperpigmentation. While a pigment-specific laser may improve the condition, sometimes the skin actually gets darker. To avoid this, an area of skin behind the ear or on a part of the face that is covered by hair may be tested to identify those at risk. Dark staining of the skin is also treated with bleaching and cortisone creams, alpha hydroxy acids, liquid nitrogen, and intermediate-strength chemical peels. Sometimes, strict sun avoidance and the simple passage of time are all that is needed.

Melasma—also known as chloasma or the "mask of pregnancy"—is brown discoloration of the skin that appears symmetrically on the face and is fueled by estrogen. It often occurs when a women is pregnant or taking birth control pills and is made worse by sun exposure that adds to a blotchiness on the cheeks, forehead, and upper lip. Except for patients with very light skin, pigment-specific laser treatment is unpredictable and often unsuccessful. However, even light-skinned women experience a high rate of recurrence if they continue to have elevated levels of estrogen and do not avoid sun exposure.

Nevi spilus are light brown lesions resembling café-au-lait spots with a sprinkling of confettilike dark brown speckles. Found on the trunk and extremities in 2 percent of the population, they can sometimes be treated successfully in multiple treatments with pigment-specific lasers, although there is the possibility of incomplete fading, hypo- and hyperpigmentation, or recurrence.

Dark circles under the eyes give people an unwelcome raccoonlike appearance. While poorly understood, it is thought that heredity, among other factors, plays a role in this discoloration.

And for those with type III or darker skin, dark circles are usually the result of pigment irregularities. The Q-switched pigment-specific lasers are often used to treat this condition, after which daily use of sunscreen and sunglasses are recommended to prevent recurrence. Sunblocks and sun-protective goggles must be worn on ski slopes because the white snow reflects onto the face, causing the dark circles to return.

Nevi of Ota and Ito. Nevus of Ota is a benign skin blemish found on the face and in or around the eye. Nevus of Ito, also benign, is usually found on the shoulder or upper arms. Both are collections of pigment in the dermis, similar in appearance to the Mongolian spots seen at the base of the spine in newborns. Because these nevi involve pigments deep in the skin, they appear as brown to grayish-blue discolorations. Under a microscope, in fact, they are similar to tattoo particles, thus making them very responsive to the light of the Q-switched pigment-specific laser systems. Before laser technology was available, there was little to offer people who were born with these nevi, which are more common in females of Asian decent. Nevi of Ota were particularly devastating, requiring excision and grafting, dermabrasion, or any other method of destroying the pigment. But these treatments also damaged the skin and created scarring and pigment alterations. Q-switched pigment-specific lasers can now eliminate these discolorations, often with no scarring or permanent pigment changes. Typically, from four to eight treatment sessions, lasting just a few minutes, are needed, with each treatment spaced about two months apart. People with darker complexions are less responsive to treatment because the light of the laser is absorbed by the first pigment it comes in contact with, which is usually the melanin found in the epidermis that competes with and prevails over the deeper melanin found in nevi of Ota and Ito. Consequently, additional treatments may be needed.

Unwanted tattoos. An estimated ten million people in the United States have at least one tattoo, and more than half want them removed! Although Pamela Anderson changed the tattoo on her ring finger from "Tommy" to "Mommy," most people who are displeased with their tattoos want them banished altogether. That includes everyone from the woman happily married to a Billy who wants the heart-encircled Jerry that she had tattooed when she was eighteen removed to the prominent attorney who wants the tattooed serpent coiling up his arm from his biker days taken off.

If a tattoo is comprised of different colors, several lasers are commonly used to target each ink's particular absorption characteristics. The lighter one's skin, the more successful the procedure will be because the melanin in darker skin competes with the laser's beam, making the light less likely to reach the deeper levels of tattoo pigment. The most stubborn tattoos, etched professionally, contain a greater amount of pigment than those etched by amateurs. Q-switched pigment-specific lasers effectively remove tattoos, Q-switching being the ability of the laser to store units of light until high-peak power is reached and then to deliver very short pulses of light at intensities that shatter tattoo inks into microscopic fragments. With each zap of the laser, a pearl-sized area of skin immediately whitens and sometimes pinpoint bleeding occurs.

When a large tattoo is lased, as many as one hundred small dots may appear alongside each other. Small white splattering flecks of skin debris are collected in the cone-shaped handpiece attached to the laser. As treatment progresses and the amount of tattoo ink dissipates, fewer tissue fragments are collected. Other fragments are engulfed and digested by the cells of the immune system that cart them off to the blood and lymphatic systems where they are promptly transported out of the body. After treatment, there may be some swelling and redness in the surrounding skin, but after a few hours the whitened dots become red and start to crust, forming small scabs. Following the procedure, antibiotic ointment and a nonstick dressing are applied. When the dressing is changed over the next several

laser tattoo removal

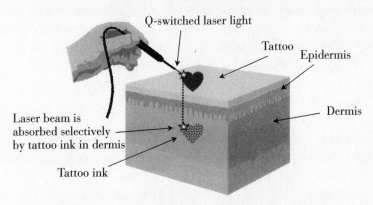

Q-switched laser light

Tattoo

Epidermis

Dermis

Laser beam is absorbed selectively by tattoo ink in dermis

Tattoo ink

The laser shatters the tattoo ink into tiny fragments, which are removed gradually by the body's immune system.

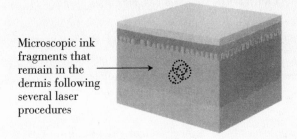

Microscopic ink fragments that remain in the dermis following several laser procedures

Normal skin is not affected during Q-switched laser treatment. Tattoo is removed and healthy tissue is left unharmed.

days, it is not unusual to see fragments of tattoo pigment being shed.

Usually the procedure is performed without the need for anesthesia or only the application of EMLA cream beforehand. The first few treatments may be uncomfortable because a great amount of tattoo ink is absorbing the laser's light, but as the pigment decreases, so does the discomfort. Generally, people report less discomfort from the laser treatment than from the original tattooing. Laser treatment may take only a few minutes if the tattoo is small but up to a half hour if it is large. On average, four to eight treatment sessions at six- to eight-week intervals are needed, but very resistant tattoos may require ten or more treatments. Even after multiple treatments, however, trace pigments may still be visible.

---

which laser will remove my tattoo?

LASER	TATTOO COLORS REMOVED
Q-switched ruby	All colors except red, orange, yellow
Q-switched alexandrite	All colors except red, orange, yellow
Q-switched Nd:YAG	All colors except red, orange, yellow, green
Q-switched frequency-doubled Nd:YAG	Red, orange, yellow
Pulsed dye laser (pigmented)	Red, orange, yellow

Unwanted permanent makeup. There are a variety of reasons why women have permanent makeup applied, and an equal number of reasons why they want it removed, including simply getting tired of it, feeling the look is out of fashion, or never having liked it in the first place. The pigments, equipment, and techniques used for micropigmentation (permanent makeup) are similar to those used by professional tattoo artists, and the technique for removing cosmetic tattoos is the same as for removing decorative tattoos, as is the follow-up care. But treating certain cosmetic tattoos with a pigment-specific laser can be risky because in removing flesh-tone colors like tan, beige, light pink, light brown, rust, and white, the iron compound ferric oxide in the tattoo can suddenly change chemically to ferrous oxide and the tattoo, paradoxically, will turn jet black, thus becoming unsightly and harder to remove. If this happens, multiple treatments may help lighten the color of the tattoo, but in some cases it may be permanent, and the only solution is complete excision or vaporization of the skin with a resurfacing laser. For removing permanent eyeliner or eyebrow makeup that does not contain the colors mentioned above, a pigment-specific laser is highly effective.

We've all looked in the mirror and remarked: "Where did *that* come from!" In less time than it takes to say "Out, damned spot! Out I say!" you can get rid of the damned spot in literally a fraction of a second, leaving the rest of your lunch break for lunch.

CHAPTER TWELVE

nonablative lasers for wrinkles

*including the CoolTouch that rejuvenates the
skin and diminishes wrinkles and acne scars*

The clinically intimidating word *ablation* refers to any surgical procedure that involves excision, or cutting into. *Nonablative* refers to a nonsurgical procedure that allows laser light to zero in on the underlying layers of skin by harmlessly bypassing the upper layers. Sort of like Casper the Friendly Ghost walking through doors and walls without causing them any harm! For untold numbers of people, nonablative laser treatment is a godsend.

Take Elizabeth, a twenty-nine-year-old newsanchor at a small TV station in the Midwest. While admitting to "as much vanity as the next person who knows how merciless the camera can be," she relied on layers of cover-up makeup to hide the leftover acne scars from her teens and the teeny-tiny fine lines that she had already begun noticing around her eyes and mouth. "I'd do anything, including nothing at all," she said, "to avoid the pain I'd heard about from all that scraping and sanding that people have on their skin."

She was alluding not only to dermabrasion but also to the deep chemical peels that have been used traditionally to burn away layers of the skin with an acid solution of, typically, either phenol or trichoroacetic acid, and that also required at least two weeks of recovery in which the treated skin sloughs off and is replaced with a new layer of revitalized skin.

Elizabeth read her share of women's magazines, but in scrambling to reach the top in her profession had somehow missed the quantum leaps in cosmetic enhancement that have evolved since the mid-1990s, when the ultra-pulsed CO_2 and erbium:YAG lasers were developed for skin resurfacing. In addition to replacing the options of deep chemical peeling or dermabrasion, these lasers worked by vaporizing the surface layer of cells, giving surgeons an added measure of control and making the procedure safer and its outcome more predictable. However, in spite of the incredible results that they yielded, there was still the problem of postprocedure discomfort and a relatively long recovery time.

Enter the nonablative lasers like CoolTouch, an Nd:YAG laser, which is the newest, coolest technique for skin rejuvenation, tightening and improving the texture of the complexion without ever wounding the surface of the skin. While nonablative lasers don't provide the dramatic results of the CO_2 or erbium lasers, they nevertheless result in visible improvement. An added advantage is that they are often offered in a series of four to six treatments of only fifteen minutes each—perfect for that lunch break!

Elizabeth usually ran from her job to the gym and then to meet and spend "as much time as possible" with her fiancé, Brian, an industrial-equipment salesman, all of which, ironically, left her almost no time to watch television. But she did catch a segment on one of the TV magazine shows that featured the pros and cons of nonablative skin resurfacing. "That was it!" she said, as she immediately began fantasizing about "the new me."

questions and answers about nonablative laser resurfacing

WHAT IS NONABLATIVE LASER RESURFACING?
Also called laser toning or subsurface resurfacing, this procedure uses a minimally invasive laser such as the CoolTouch to directly target water and collagen in the deeper layer of skin without any wounding, burning, or peeling of the overlying skin. Nonablative laser resurfacing encourages the growth of new collagen, thus improving the appearance of wrinkles, acne scars, and chicken pox scars.

WHO IS A CANDIDATE?
The ideal candidate for CoolTouch is looking for facial rejuvenation but cannot afford the downtime that is needed for the more aggressive treatments and dramatic results that dermabrasion, deep chemical peels, or the CO_2 and erbium lasers provide. While the results of CoolTouch treatments, particularly for wrinkle removal, are subtler, they nonetheless result in an improvement in skin texture and an overall healthy appearance. The treatments are safe and effective on all pigmentation and skin types. Those who typically achieve the best results from CoolTouch have shallow indented acne and chicken pox scars, just the beginning of fine lines on the face, a slight loss of skin tone, minimal sun damage—and realistic expectations. The very best results are realized in relatively young adults, possibly because they have healthier fibroblasts, which are the cells that produce collagen, and in those with Fitzpatrick skin types I, II, or III. (See Chapter 2, "Your Skin, the Sun, and Your Lifestyle.")

ARE THERE ALTERNATIVES TO NONABLATIVE LASER REJUVENATION?

Resurfacing the skin with the CO_2 or erbium laser in a single session is far more effective *if* you can afford about two weeks of downtime until your skin is fully healed and approximately two to three months until the pinkness completely fades away.

HOW DO I PREPARE FOR THE PROCEDURE?

Avoid the sun or take proper precautions by applying sunscreen and wearing a hat. If you have a history of herpes cold sores, you will be prescribed a prophylactic antiviral medication to avoid a flare-up.

WHAT ARE THE TIMING OPTIONS FOR THIS PROCEDURE?

Generally, treatments are scheduled on a monthly basis, but sometimes more or less frequently, depending on the condition of your skin.

HOW IS THE PROCEDURE PERFORMED?

You will be given plastic goggles to protect your eyes from the laser light. Immediately before each pulse of the laser is emitted, your skin is cooled with a brief burst of cryogen spray. Amazingly, the beam of light passes through the overlying epidermis and goes directly to the collagen-producing cells in the underlying dermis. During the procedure, a sensor measures the temperature of your skin in order to determine the appropriate dosage of the laser's light. The goal is to elevate the temperature in the dermis to 80° centigrade in order to stimulate the production of new collagen, which continues to generate for two to three months.

WILL I NEED AN ANESTHETIC?

Approximately an hour before the procedure, it is helpful to numb your skin by applying EMLA or a similar topical anesthetic that your dermatologist or plastic surgeon can recommend.

HOW WILL I LOOK IMMEDIATELY AFTER?

Your skin will be pink and flushed and appear as if you had just worked out at the gym, and your face may be slightly swollen. But no bandages are required since the treatment leaves no wounds, no bleeding, and no crusting. You can apply moisturizer, sunscreen, and makeup and return to work immediately or plan to go out to dinner in the evening. In about two hours, the pinkness and swelling will subside.

HOW WILL I FEEL IMMEDIATELY AFTER?

Your face might sting a bit, but not to the point that you won't feel comfortable returning to your normal life.

HOW LONG DOES THE PROCEDURE TAKE?

From fifteen to thirty minutes from beginning to end.

HOW MANY TREATMENTS WILL I REQUIRE?

From four to six. After a single treatment, it takes about one to three months to notice visible results, including a more youthful appearance with fewer wrinkles and less obvious scars. But results vary from patient to patient depending on age, skin type, and the condition of the skin. Most people follow their initial series of treatments with a maintenance program in order to continue to retard the effects of aging and to avoid more aggressive treatment such as ablative laser resurfacing or a facelift.

WHAT DOES THE RECOVERY ENTAIL?

No postprocedure care is necessary other than scrupulously avoiding the sun.

WHAT ARE THE RISKS?

When CoolTouch technology was introduced, some patients developed blisters, scabs, crusting, or even pitted scars after the procedure. New and improved machines have all but done away with these postprocedure problems.

ARE THERE ANY SPECIAL CONCERNS FOR WOMEN OF COLOR?

People of color are vulnerable to postinflammatory hypopigmentation (lightening of the skin) or hyperpigmentation (darkening of the skin through an overproduction of melanin) because their skin is rich in pigmentation. Fortunately, the newer machines allow doctors to cool the skin both immediately before and after the procedure, making the treatment safer for people of all skin types.

WILL PEOPLE BE ABLE TO TELL THAT I HAD NONABLATIVE LASER RESURFACING?

Immediately after the procedure, any swelling or pinkness can be covered up with makeup, so it's unlikely that anyone will notice any changes. However, as the days and weeks elapse, the appearance of wrinkles and acne scars will diminish as your skin gradually heals from the inside, restoring a more youthful appearance to your face. It's quite probable that you'll be hearing people tell you how terrific you look.

WHAT DO NONABLATIVE LASER TREATMENTS COST?

If a medical doctor performs the treatment, the cost is between $500 and $1,000 per session. If a physician's assistant, nurse practitioner, or registered nurse performs the procedure, the cost is approximately $400 per session.

ARE THERE OTHER NONABLATIVE LASERS OR LIGHT SOURCES THAT CAN ACHIEVE SIMILAR RESULTS?

Full-face treatments using an intense pulsed light can be used to treat patients who have hyperpigmentation, lax skin, freckles, early sunspots, large pores, fine lines, a ruddy complexion, and broken blood vessels. After the first treatment, new collagen begins to form in the skin, smoothing its texture, making the pores appear smaller and diminishing fine lines and wrinkles. The treatments require no downtime, and after a series of treatments, many patients say that they look five years younger! Names of the intense pulsed light treatments include IPL Facial, FotoFacial, PhotoFacial, Photorejuvenation, and EpiFacial.

Other popular nonablative resurfacing lasers include the SmoothBeam and the N-Lite. The SmoothBeam is a skin-remodeling diode laser that allows physicians to offer nonablative skin-renewal services at a fraction of the cost of competing laser systems because the manufacturer, Candela, responding to the pressures that managed care has placed on doctors to sustain or increase their incomes, has made it available to 110,000 physicians in the United States—including gynecologists, ophthalmologists, and general practitioners—instead of to only the 15,000 doctors who practice dermatology and plastic surgery. While physicians who don't specialize in skin care can certainly use this laser system, it behooves every patient to ask the right questions and guard against practitioners who have minimal knowledge or experience. (See Chapter 4, "Better Safe Than Sorry.")

The N-Lite, a pulsed-dye laser, is the first selective nonablative laser system cleared by the FDA for reducing wrinkles around the eyes and is therefore quite popular with ophthalmologists. The N-Lite targets the blood vessels beneath the skin's surface to stimulate new collagen formation, which reduces the depth of wrinkles. Like other nonablative laser systems, the outcome of a series of treatments varies from subtle to clearly visible improvement.

IS ANY SPECIAL TRAINING REQUIRED TO PERFORM THIS PROCEDURE?

Usually, dermatologists and plastic surgeons administer nonablative laser treatments. However, physician assistants, nurse practitioners, and registered nurses can perform the procedure if supervised by a medical doctor. (See Chapter 4, "Better Safe Than Sorry.")

WHAT IS THE SATISFACTION RATE FROM THIS PROCEDURE?

It is not uncommon for patients to be more excited about this procedure than their doctors! This may be because doctors who perform cosmetic procedures are sometimes greater perfectionists than those patients who are more than willing to sacrifice perfection to the lower cost and virtual absence of downtime that this technique offers.

In addition, many doctors prefer to hit a grand slam by performing a single aggressive procedure that obviates the necessity of return trips. But increasing numbers of patients are happy simply to get on first base with a less dramatic but quite satisfying lunchtime quick fix. In fact, many believe that several base hits add up to a home run!

laser treatment of unwanted hair

on the upper lip, chin, bikini area, underarms, and everyplace else

It's well known that women are obsessed with the hair on their heads—the length, cut, style, and color. One of their greatest fears is the dreaded "bad hair day." Less publicized is their obsession with unwanted hair elsewhere. After all, what woman wants to admit that she has a mustache or—horrors!—a beard? Yet in the privacy of their bathrooms, many women search for and pluck, bleach, shave, or wax away unwanted hair from all parts of their bodies.

Bianca is a perfect example. The stunning twenty-eight-year-old pop singer had inherited her sparkling personality and powerful voice from her father, a real estate salesman and also an Irish tenor who sang first as a choirboy in church, in a traveling barbershop quartet as a teenager, and in community theater musical comedies as an adult. From her mother, a native of Mexico, Bianca had inherited a sense of fierce determination, statuesque good looks, an olive complexion, and—the bane of her life—hair there and everywhere.

Even before her teens, Bianca started plucking her eyebrows, bleaching the hair above her lips, and shaving her legs. By the age of fourteen, she was getting bikini and arm waxes. And in college, she was spending several hours a week in an off-campus salon having hair removed from all the old places and some new ones, like her face and abdomen.

"I was a slave," she said. "When my friends used to discuss what subjects they planned to major in, I used to think to myself, 'I'm already majoring—in getting rid of my hair!'" When she quit school in her junior year to pursue singing, the problem became worse.

"When you're under a spotlight, everything is magnified," she explained. "I loved the midriff look but hated to wear it. I was so self-conscious thinking that some of my stubble was showing that I seriously thought about quitting and getting a job developing pictures in a darkroom!"

Fate intervened when on the way to one of her many trips to the "waxing witch," as Bianca called the woman who peeled away her body hair every week, she heard a radio ad for laser hair removal, with its tantalizing promise to "be hair-free and carefree!" Making a U-turn, she headed straight toward the dermatologist's office. The doctor explained the benefits of removing hair with a laser but warned her, "If you think this system means hair today, gone tomorrow, you'll be disappointed!"

Undaunted, Bianca signed the consent form immediately. Within months, she was wearing a diamond (well, actually zircon) stud in her navel and singing her heart out.

questions and answers about laser hair removal

WHAT SHOULD I KNOW ABOUT LASER HAIR REMOVAL?

Among other things, that it has improved dramatically over the past few years. In 1995, the FDA approved SoftLight, the first laser hair removal system that used a Q-switched Nd:YAG laser along with a special carbon solution. The procedure involved waxing, immediately followed by the application of a black carbon solution that was massaged into the skin so that it could concentrate in empty pores and penetrate to the deepest level of the hair follicles. The laser then zapped the solution, heating and expanding the carbon pigment until it exploded and shattered, effectively disabling the hair follicle. The messy solution has since been done away with, relegated to the trash bin of medical gimmicks. The whole procedure proved to be no more effective than waxing alone.

A few years after the Nd:YAG's debut, several companies received FDA approval to use other light sources for hair removal, the most common being the long-pulsed ruby and alexandrite lasers, the diode laser, and an intense pulsed light source. You may not know these systems by their generic names but you've certainly seen their brand names advertised: Cool-Glide, Epilaser, GentleLASE, LightSheer, and EpiLight.

Major breakthroughs in improving the effectiveness and safety of laser hair removal include the development of chilling devices to cool the overlying epidermis and longer pulse durations that allow the beam of light to penetrate more deeply into the hair follicles without harming the overlying skin.

HOW DOES LASER HAIR REMOVAL WORK?

Laser is an acronym for light amplification by stimulated emission of radiation, which in English means that it produces highly concentrated beams of light to destroy particular targets. In hair removal, the laser beam passes through the epidermis, zeroing in on the pigment (melanin) surrounding the hair. The pigment selectively absorbs the laser's energy and the hair follicle is damaged, thus preventing it from producing hair in the near future and leaving the skin smooth and hairless. According to the FDA, "permanent" simply means eradicating the unwanted hair for longer than six months. After treatment, hair grows back finer and lighter, but it stills grows back, which is why manufacturers claim that their hair-removal lasers achieve permanent hair *reduction*, and not permanent *removal*.

WHO IS A CANDIDATE?

Prime candidates used to be only people with white skin and dark hair, but advances have translated into a greater safety pro-

laser hair removal

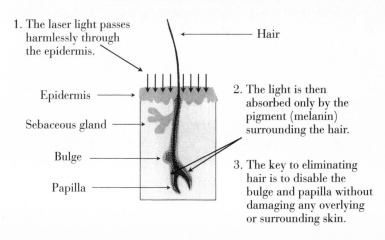

1. The laser light passes harmlessly through the epidermis.

Hair

Epidermis

Sebaceous gland

Bulge

Papilla

2. The light is then absorbed only by the pigment (melanin) surrounding the hair.

3. The key to eliminating hair is to disable the bulge and papilla without damaging any overlying or surrounding skin.

file for those with darker complexions, including Indians, Asians, Hispanics, and those of Middle Eastern and Mediterranean ancestry. It is extremely important, however, for darker-skinned people to request that state-of-the-art technology be used for laser hair removal to avoid the lightening or darkening of the skin and possible burning, scabbing, and scarring that may result if older machines are used.

Laser hair removal is effective only on dark coarse hair, not the blond peach fuzz variety that most people have on their faces. The procedure will not work on people who have blond or gray hair because laser light is not attracted to—indeed, cannot "see"—its pigments. Women commonly request that their upper lip, chin, bikini line, underarms, and legs be treated. Men, who comprise about 15 percent of those seeking hair removal, want to get rid of the hair on their backs and chests.

HOW DO I PREPARE FOR MY PROCEDURE?

Before laser hair removal, strictly avoid sun exposure and self-tanners. On the day of treatment, wear loose-fitting clothes and do not apply makeup to any area being treated. Try not to wax or tweeze immediately before the procedure because the hair needs to be in the follicle in order to attract the laser's beam of light. But you can shave or use a depilatory that removes hair only above the surface of the skin.

HOW IS THE PROCEDURE PERFORMED?

As with all laser procedures, the eyes are protected with goggles. The skin is gently cleansed, and if there is significant hair growth in the area to be treated, it is shaved. It is never waxed or plucked because these methods take hair from the roots, which prevents the laser beam from reaching its target: the skin pigment that surrounds the roots. As the beam of light sweeps over the skin, the tiny amount of remaining stubble is zapped, often creating an odor that is similar to fresh-popped popcorn. In certain laser systems, a cool gel protects the overlying epidermis from injury; in others the laser handpiece has a built-in chill tip or cooling spray.

CAN LASER HAIR REMOVAL BE USED TO MANAGE INGROWN HAIRS?

Yes. Many men, particularly men of color, have ingrown hairs on their faces or necks called pseudofolliculitis barbae. After a few treatments the shaving bumps subside. Since the hair grows back more slowly and finely, the condition improves greatly.

WILL I NEED AN ANESTHETIC?

Most people say that the laser sensation feels like pinpricks, tingles from a sparkler, a burst of heat, or a sting. Those with a low pain threshold or who are having hair removed in sensitive areas can apply EMLA cream beforehand or the doctor can numb the areas with lidocaine. But with newer methods of chilling the overlying skin, laser hair removal has become quite tolerable.

HOW WILL I LOOK IMMEDIATELY AFTER?

Your skin may be slightly flushed with some mottling or welts, but there will be no crusting or bruising. Sometimes a prickly heat rash or inflammation around the hair follicles (folliculitis) may occur and is treated with mild steroid cream or topical antibiotic lotion. Makeup can be applied after a couple of hours.

HOW LONG DOES THE PROCEDURE TAKE?

The upper lip may take only a few minutes, a man's entire back about thirty minutes, and the legs about one to two hours, depending on the speed of the laser system that is used.

WHAT DOES THE RECOVERY ENTAIL?

Nothing! After a few hours of transient mottled pinkness and mild swelling, your skin will be smooth, soft, and hair-free, at least for a while. With some laser systems it takes several days to a week for the injured hair to fall out. Avoid sunlight as well as skin lotions and oils that contain fragrances for a few days because the skin will be sensitive and more vulnerable to irritation.

HOW LONG WILL THE RESULTS LAST?

Factors like your age, gender, ethnicity, hormone levels, and the body area that is treated are all variables that determine the rate of hair growth—and regrowth. A woman who has hair removed from her bikini area or legs may find herself hair-free for the entire summer, but hair removed from her upper lip starts to return after just a few weeks. The thick, coarse chin hairs seem to be the most stubborn, probably because hormones greatly influence their growth; it may take six or eight treatments to disable them. Conversely, hairs in the bikini area seem the most responsive to treatment. Depending on the individual, treatments are usually given at one- to four-month intervals. As they progress, the time that a person remains relatively hair-free is longer. As with hair dying, frosting, or bleaching, those who desire a greater freedom from unwanted hair must have periodic follow-up treatments.

ARE THERE ANY LIMITATIONS OR RISKS?

Anyone who has had laser resurfacing, dermabrasion, or a deep chemical peel, all of which sensitize the skin, should wait several months before having laser hair removal in the facial area.

Those who are using Accutane must delay treatment until the medication has been discontinued for six months.

Hair removal on the upper lip must be delayed if cold sores are present.

Flare-ups of psoriasis, lupus, or other inflammatory conditions preclude laser hair removal.

Women with abnormal hair growth *may* have a hormonal imbalance and should be evaluated by a physician to rule out ovarian or adrenal gland disorders or other endocrine gland problems. While it is safe to perform laser hair removal if an underlying hormonal condition exists, a correct diagnosis and treatment might obviate the need for the procedure.

People who have been treated with gold therapy for arthritis should not have laser hair removal because microscopic remnants of gold may remain in the skin, and the areas of skin treated with laser light may turn black. The same is true of those who have had permanent makeup containing white or red pigments applied. (See Chapter 11, "Laser Treatment of Brown Blemishes.")

Hyperpigmentation and hypopigmentation are not uncommon, and scarring can occur if proper laser safety precautions are not taken.

A note of caution: A number of malpractice lawsuits have been waged by patients whose skin has been burned during laser hair removal. Yet in many states, laser hair removal is performed in spas and salons by aestheticians, electrologists, and nurses who are *not* under the direct supervision of a medical doctor.

Dermatologists argue that their knowledge of the skin and their ability to diagnose and treat hormonal problems that may cause abnormal hair growth, as well as their ability to deal with complications, make them better qualified than nonphysicians to perform laser procedures. Fifteen states do not allow anyone other than a physician to perform laser hair removal, and many states require a physician's direct supervision. (See Chapter 4, "Better Safe Than Sorry.")

WHAT DOES THE PROCEDURE COST?

The market for laser hair removal has exploded in the last few years with many physicians as well as beauty salons and spas offering the procedure. Because of the competition, more afford-able laser systems are being sold and the fees have come down significantly. Removing hair from the upper lip, chin, arms, or bikini area costs approximately $250 for each individual site per session. When multiple areas are treated, discounts are usually offered, and since significant hair reduction usually requires several treatments, "package deals" are commonplace.

ARE THERE ALTERNATIVES TO THE PROCEDURE?

While laser hair removal is the most efficient and effective method to get rid of unwanted hair, other methods are still help-ful in some cases.

Bleaching is not actually a method of hair removal but it makes unwanted hair less apparent. Most hair bleaches contain hydrogen peroxide and ammonia that lighten hair but may irri-tate the skin.

Shaving with a razor blade or electric shaver is the age-old method of temporarily removing the hair shafts that peek out of the skin. No matter how you cut it—or shave it—most women hate the stubble. Although few have enough facial hair to experi-ence a five o'clock shadow, there are women who shave their faces and are deeply embarrassed by their facial hair growth.

However, despite the widespread belief that shaving increases hair growth or makes the hair grow back thicker, no data support this notion.

Waxing involves the application of hot wax to areas of unwanted hair growth. After the wax is applied, it is rapidly pulled off with a cloth, taking with it not only the hairs but also often the top layers of the epidermis. Ouch!

Sugaring kits made from water and sugar or honey work like wax but they wash off easily and are less abrasive on sensitive areas like the upper lip.

Plucking hairs with a tweezer is usually reserved for limited areas of the body such as the eyebrows, upper lip, or stray hairs on the chin or around the nipple.

Chemical depilatories like Nair or Neet are topical agents that soften the hair shaft until it is dissolved by a chemical reaction. While tolerable to some women, they often have offensive odors and can be extremely irritating on sensitive skin.

Electrolysis is a slow, tedious, painful, and invasive hair-by-hair removal process in which a weak electrical current is passed through a tiny needle into the depth of the hair follicle. As the hot current zaps away, hot sodium hydroxide (lye) is produced that destroys each follicle. Satisfying results, which take months of weekly visits, are totally dependent on the skill of the operator. A client must also trust the sterility of the equipment and be aware that a needle used in several sites has the potential to spread wart or herpes viruses and other blood-borne pathogens. In addition, the electric needle my cause scarring. In contrast, laser hair removal is so efficient and rapid that large areas such as the entire upper lip, the chin, or armpit can be treated in a ten-minute session without the risk of contamination or scarring.

Threading uses a thin thread that is manipulated rapidly to remove hair from the face, arms, and other areas of the body.

Vaniqa (eflornithine hydrochloride) is not actually a method of hair removal. It is the first prescription cream that slows the growth of unwanted facial hair in women by blocking a key enzyme in hair production. In clinical trials, approximately 50 percent of women reported significant slowing of the rate of regrowth after using the cream for six months. The cream's effects become visible after twice-a-day applications for one or two months, and it can be used in conjunction with any method of hair removal. The cream has been approved by the FDA for use on the face but doctors are already prescribing it for off-label use on the bikini line and around the nipples. The net effect is prolonged intervals between the need to remove hair. However, once you stop applying Vaniqa, your hair grows back at the same rate as it did before. For many women, a tube of Vaniqa that costs about $50 and lasts about two to three months is well worth the money.

Laser hair removal is light-years ahead of any other method. Fees have come down and the popularity of the procedure is at an all-time high. If you have unwanted facial or body hair, throw away your tweezers and forget about the other Marquis de Sade procedures. A few lunchtime laser breaks and you'll wonder how you put up with the old-time hair-removal methods for so long.

laser treatment of red problems

for broken blood vessels, rosacea,
spider angiomas, port-wine stains,
and stretch marks

The menu was "typical Katrina," her friends said. Having dined at her quirkily decorated apartment numerous times, they were accustomed to not even guessing what she was going to serve. The last feast was prepared while Katrina was going through her Picasso "blue period" phase. As a vintage recording of Oscar Levant playing "Rhapsody in Blue" filled the air, Katrina served predinner snacks of blue corn tortilla chips, an appetizer of bluepoint oysters, an entrée of bluefish, blue curaçao to drink, and blueberries for dessert. The table, of course, was decorated with delphiniums and blue hydrangeas.

When her friends arrived for the latest sit-down, they didn't know what to expect. Katrina, who was a thirty-four-year-old sous chef at a popular Key West eatery and, by any measure, a free spirit, never failed to surprise—even thrill—the people she invited to dine with her. Sure enough, the table looked beautiful, awash with red roses, poppies, and carnations.

"Gaugin!" one friend guessed as he looked over the mouthwatering color of the moment. There were sumptuous-looking lobsters, salads of tomatoes and red peppers, what seemed like gallons of Bloody Marys, and piles of cherries and strawberries. In the background, "Lady in Red" was playing, followed by "Red Red Wine" and songs sung by Sammy Hagar, King Crimson, Tara Maclean, Heaven 17, Sister Soleil, Belly, Dirty Three, and Naked—all with the title "Red."

Usually, Katrina expounded on her dinner themes, but this time she made her friends guess. "Anger?" No. "Passion?" No. "A fire sale?" No. "We give up!" one of the group said.

"I'm celebrating!" Katrina exclaimed, putting her face up to the light to reveal skin that was atypically smooth, nonflushed, and without any of the little pink bumps and whiteheads around her cheeks and nose that had made her self-conscious since her early twenties.

Her friends were impressed and told her so. They listened as Katrina explained that she had just learned that her condition had a name, rosacea, and that it had to do with the red pigment in her broken blood vessels. "Now there's a special laser that can zap the blood vessels in only five or ten minutes," she explained, "and it took only three treatments for me to get rid of this scourge.

"The celebration," she told them, "is because now I love the color red, as long as it's not on my face!"

questions and answers about vascular-specific laser treatment

WHO IS A CANDIDATE FOR VASCULAR-SPECIFIC LASER TREATMENT OF RED PROBLEMS?

Anyone who has small vascular (vein) imperfections and dilated or broken blood vessels that appear as chronically pink and red areas around the corners of the nose and on the cheeks is a candidate for vascular-specific laser treatment. These fragile, linear, spiderlike vessels, called telangiectasias, which are common in people with fair, sensitive skin (types I and II), can "break" from overzealous use of Buf-Pufs or other exfoliants as well as from mechanical irritation from washing, scrubbing, or squeezing blackheads and pimples. In addition, Retin-A, sun exposure, chronic use of steroid creams on the face, and any kind of nasal surgery such as rhinoplasty (a nose job) can worsen the situation. People with lupus, scleroderma, or other connective tissue diseases, who are more prone to prominent facial blood vessels, are candidates, as are those with rosacea, a red birthmark like a port-wine stain, an acquired red mark such as a spider angioma, and pink stretch marks and scars.

HOW DOES THE VASCULAR-SPECIFIC LASER WORK ON BROKEN BLOOD VESSELS?

The laser's beam of light passes through the skin as though the skin were invisible and selectively targets the red pigment in the bloodstream (hemoglobin) that lies within the vessels. The heat of the laser beam coagulates the blood and destroys the blood vessel walls without breaking or damaging the overlying skin.

laser treatment for broken blood vessels

Excess broken blood vessels
in the upper dermis.

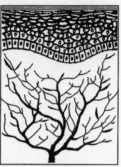

1. Laser light heats and
seals excess blood vessels.

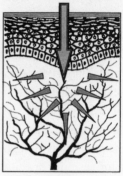

2. White blood cells remove
fragments of the sealed laser-
treated blood vessels.

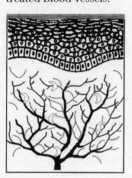

3. Normal blood vessels
are restored.

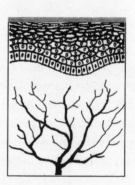

HOW DO I PREPARE FOR MY PROCEDURE?

Simply avoid the sun before treatment, which ensures that
melanin, the color-bearing pigment in the skin, does not compete
with or distract the beam of light from zeroing in on the red pigment in the blood of the vessels below.

HOW IS THE PROCEDURE PERFORMED?

The technique varies depending on the vascular laser that your doctor uses. In the case of the pulsed dye laser, rapid pulses are delivered along the course of the blood vessel, laying down a strand of pearl-sized dots that cause immediate bruising. When an area of diffuse redness is treated, such as the cheek or nose, the entire network of dilated capillaries is lased in one session as the doctor "connects the dots" until the area appears totally purple. Newer, improved pulsed dye lasers like the Vbeam or Sclerolaser cause much less bruising than earlier models, and vascular-specific lasers like the VersaPulse or light sources like the Photoderm may cause no bruising at all.

HOW LONG DOES THE PROCEDURE TAKE?

Just a few minutes.

WILL I NEED AN ANESTHETIC?

Probably not. Most adults are able to tolerate the mild sensations of laser zaps, which feel like a rubber band snapping against the skin in the case of the pulsed dye laser. With the VersaPulse, it feels like a pin being dragged along the skin. Applying the topical anesthetic EMLA cream an hour before a treatment session can numb the skin, but it can also constrict the blood vessels and diminish the effects of the treatment.

HOW WILL I LOOK IMMEDIATELY AFTER?

In the case of the pulsed dye laser, you will probably have some bruising that may last for up to ten days, but it can be immediately covered with a concealer or foundation makeup. Less bruising occurs when alternative lasers and light sources are used.

HOW MANY TREATMENTS WILL I NEED?

After a single treatment you will see definite improvement, but usually a few sessions are needed for optimal results.

WHAT DOES THE RECOVERY ENTAIL?

No posttreatment care is necessary other than covering any bruising or discoloration with camouflage makeup. Sometimes, vitamin K cream may be prescribed to hasten the healing of the bruises. Of course, avoiding sun exposure is a must! The skin of the treated areas is more sensitive after treatment and if you get a tan, hyperpigmentation (a temporary staining or browning of the skin) may develop in these areas.

HOW LONG WILL THE RESULTS LAST?

The improvement may last for years *if* you avoid products like Renova and Retin-A that are known to increase blood vessel formation. Also, avoid harsh scrubbing of the face, overuse of Buf-Pufs and other exfoliants, alcohol, spicy foods, and sun exposure.

ARE THERE ANY LIMITATIONS OR RISKS?

The greatest limitations are temporary bruising, which fades, and temporary hyperpigmentation, which usually goes away on its own in a few weeks. Since the advent of longer pulsed lasers and the use of cooling techniques, postprocedure bruising is significantly diminished, although it can still happen. Occasionally, hypopigmentation (lightening of the skin) or a subtle indentation of the skin occurs temporarily. There is a very low risk of permanent scarring.

WHAT DOES THE PROCEDURE COST?

The cost may be several hundred dollars or more, depending on the size of the area and the number of treatments required.

WHICH CONDITIONS CAN BE TREATED WITH VASCULAR-SPECIFIC LASERS?

Rosacea, a chronic condition involving involuntary flushing and blushing of the central portion of the face, affects fourteen million Americans, most of them women in their thirties or forties. While its origins are unknown, it is thought to have a genetic basis and is more common in people with fair skin and light eyes and those of Irish, English, or Scandinavian descent. About 10 percent of Swedes have the disorder. Princess Diana suffered from the condition as well. Rosacea often worsens after exposure to sun or wind, exercise, hot baths, drinking alcohol or hot beverages, and eating spicy foods. In addition to broken blood vessels, rosacea is often characterized by tiny pink bumps and whiteheads around the cheeks and nose.

Treatment often includes oral antibiotics like tetracycline, topical antibiotics, mild steroids, and topical medications like MetroGel and Noritate cream (metronidazole) or those containing sulfur. Metronidazole kills mites that often colonize on the skin of people who have increased sebum (oil) production, such as those with rosacea. The drug also diminishes inflammation and redness and is helpful in treating the little pimples and pustules that sometimes occur. Many women wear green-tinted camouflage makeup to help counteract the skin's reddish appearance.

Before laser treatment, the broken blood vessels of rosacea were often treated with a fine epilating needle like that used in electrolysis, but the needle was not "photoselective." Scarring was a risk if the energy was too high, and the treatment was ineffective if it was too low. In contrast, the vascular-specific laser "sees" only the pink or red of the vessels and therefore spares the overlying epidermis any damage. Because the skin is chilled during the procedure, there is minimal discomfort and people can return to work immediately, covering up any temporary bruising with camouflage makeup.

Note: Don't confuse rosacea with "adult acne." Acne often involves the shoulders, neck, and back, while rosacea is limited to the face. Also, blackheads are commonly seen in acne but not in rosacea. The two conditions require different treatments and some acne medications can make rosacea worse.

Rhinophyma (or red-nose syndrome) is related to rosacea. It affects more men than women, particularly in middle or older age, and is especially common in people of Irish or Celtic descent. W. C. Fields and Santa Claus are famous examples of rhinophyma sufferers. The condition is characterized by a gradually enlarging reddened and misshapen nose with enlarged pores, the result of the overgrowth of skin and sebaceous glands as well as the proliferation of blood vessels. Many people with rhinophyma are assumed to have a serious alcohol problem, but alcohol does not cause the condition although it can exacerbate it. While the vascular-specific laser treats the redness, a misshapen nose may be resculpted with the CO_2 resurfacing laser.

Stretch marks, also known as striae, typically result from pregnancy, adolescent growth spurts, weight lifting, or rapid weight gain in areas that have undergone extensive stretching such as the hips, tummy, and breasts. Estrogen also seems to play a role in their development, as do high levels of steroids that are produced by the body, ingested as prednisone or anabolic steroids, or topically applied in cream or ointment form.

As the skin stretches, collagen and elastin fibers rupture and begin to appear as pink, red, or purple streaks of wrinkled skin that later become silvery white. Since heredity pretty much determines who will and will not get stretch marks, there is no

way to prevent these sources of self-consciousness and embarrassment. Cocoa butter and other potions that promise to firm the
slackened skin do little to improve the appearance of stretch
marks. Retin-A or alpha hydroxy acids used at home, as well as
microdermabrasion, are often effective when combined with
laser treatment.

Several vascular-specific laser treatments, spaced about six
to eight weeks apart, are needed to diminish pink stretch marks,
but early red stretch marks respond the best. White stretch
marks may improve in texture, but they will probably not disappear even with repeated treatments. Small stretch marks respond
better than large ones, but even with repeated treatments they
may never completely vanish. The beneficial effects of a single
treatment may not be visible for two months or longer. Before
spending a lot of money, it is wise to have a limited test area
treated first.

Scars and keloids. In genetically susceptible individuals,
raised pink scars and keloids may result from cardiac bypass
surgery, facelift surgery, ear piercing, and other operations or
trauma. Scars are flatter, lighter in color, and more pliable after
several treatments with a vascular-specific laser and they don't
itch or burn as much if at all. The laser heats the blood vessels
in the scar, causing an alteration of tissue metabolism that
brings about collagen remodeling. For optimal results, laser
treatments are often combined with injections of steroids or the
application of silicone gel dressings or Mederma gel (an onion-
derived extract that helps scarred skin appear smoother and
softer). While pink scars can be significantly improved, realistic expectations are important: the scar will never be *completely* erased.

Spider angiomas are clusters of tiny linear blood vessels
that usually emanate from a central point on the face; hence,
their spiderlike appearance. They are often seen in pregnant
women and just as often disappear spontaneously after delivery.

When not associated with pregnancy, however, they have a tendency to persist but can be zapped away in minutes with a vascular-specific laser.

Poikiloderma of Civatte gives new meaning to the term *redneck*. Characterized by a flushed, splotchy, red appearance on the sides of the neck, this condition is of unknown origin and more common in women after menopause. It is sometimes associated with a burning sensation and exacerbated by sun exposure and the use of perfumes on the neck area. Several treatments with a vascular-specific laser are needed before the redness fades. To prevent recurrence, vigilant sun protection is a must.

Port-wine stains or other red birthmarks. Not everyone is born with a port-wine stain like Gorbachev's. In fact, they are quite rare, occurring in three babies out of one thousand. This vascular malformation, which consists of a dense network of blood vessels beneath the surface of the skin on the face or neck or other body parts, affects girls and boys equally. As a person gets older and the port-wine stain matures and thickens, the stain often forms little vascular cobblestone bumps or blebs that are not only a cosmetic nuisance but also vulnerable to trauma and bleeding.

Any age person—from an infant to an adult of sixty, seventy, eighty, or beyond—is a candidate for vascular-specific laser treatment, which is quick and easy and can certainly be performed in six to ten or more sessions on a series of lunch breaks, spaced about four weeks apart. Because the pulsed dye laser is so gentle and there is such a low incidence of scarring, this form of port-wine stain removal is considered unequaled in treating infants as young as a few weeks of age. The way a particular stain responds is related to its anatomical location as well as its color. Generally, a dark flat stain located on the face or neck responds very well, while a stain on the central portion of the face, or on the forearms, hands, legs, or feet requires a greater number of treatments. Even with multiple treatments, the stain may not completely disappear, but stubborn stains may still lighten significantly to a very pale pink or salmon.

Warts. Conventional methods of wart removal as well as CO_2 laser treatment can be highly successful in destroying the wart virus, but may result in scarring. However, no scarring occurs when the pulsed dye laser zaps a wart. The laser's beam is absorbed by the wart's dilated blood vessels, and the heat of the laser destroys the wart virus. Several sessions, two to four weeks apart, are needed for wart removal, but there is no guarantee that the treatment will work. Thick, elevated warts that are covered with a callus and deep plantar warts must be pared down before laser treatment.

Miscellaneous vascular lumps and bumps. Cherry angiomas are tiny, bright red, raised bumps found mostly on the trunk and upper extremities and occur in more than 85 percent of middle-aged and elderly people. Venous lakes are small blue nodules commonly found on the lower lip, ear, or other sun-exposed areas in older people. These vascular lesions are benign and, from a medical point of view, don't need to be treated. However, if you don't like the look of them, a few simple zaps of the electrocautery machine or vascular-specific laser will remove them in seconds.

Psoriasis. This chronic inflammatory skin disorder affects five million Americans and tends to run in families, although its etiology is unknown. It causes pink- or salmon-colored scaly patches and plaques on the elbows, knees, and other parts of the body. Named for the Greek word meaning "itch," psoriasis may itch but it usually does not. The condition can be physically disfiguring and socially debilitating, causing people who believe it is contagious—which it is not—to avoid those who have it. A vascular-specific laser can be used safely along with more conventional methods such as topical steroids, vitamin D and A ointments, ultraviolet light, and various oral medications. The lesions of psoriasis contain dilated blood vessels that absorb the light of the pulsed dye laser well, but the newest and most promising laser for the treatment of psoriasis is an excimer laser. (See Chapter 5, "Quick Fixes.")

Acne. A pulsed dye laser is helpful in the treatment of inflammatory acne. The laser's beam of light selectively eliminates the small blood vessels that are associated with the condition's red pimples.

Wrinkles. Vascular-specific lasers have shown subtle improvement in the appearance of fine wrinkling, possibly by stimulating the production of new collagen and elastic tissue. (See Chapter 12, "Nonablative Lasers for Wrinkles.")

There are so many red skin problems that practically everyone, at some time in life, can benefit from a quick zap of the laser. With the new and improved treatments, you no longer have to feel self-conscious about this or that unattractive blemish. A quick detour at lunchtime to your dermatologist's or plastic surgeon's office will help you get the red out.

CHAPTER FIFTEEN

laser and other
treatments of leg veins

zapping away those unattractive
spider veins

Ann-Marie, a sexy-looking blonde whose parents and grand-parents came from northern Italy, swore that she "never ate lunch in a sitting position." The forty-five-year-old registered nurse and mother of four—all born a year apart—described an on-the-go life that began in childhood when she was a gofer and then a waitress in her parents' mom-and-pop restaurant, contin-ued when she entered nursing school at the age of eighteen, and took on marathon status when she became a mother.

"Being a waitress and working in the ER is the same thing," she said. "You never sit—*never*! And with kids, you grab a bite here, a nibble there. To this day, every time I go out to dinner with my husband, I still can't get used to sitting for two hours and actually having someone else serve *me*!"

As a nurse, Ann-Marie knew that her prominent varicose veins and the many spider veins that wended their way along her legs were the result of genes, obesity, and estrogen. "I'm the stereotype," she said. "My mother had the same problem at the same age, I'm pretty overweight and, of course, I have plenty of estrogen!"

By age fifty-five, 50 percent of women and 15 percent of men develop varicose veins, which are a superficial network of vessels that result from faulty valves that cause vessels to dilate and blood to stagnate. Aggravating factors include pregnancy, trauma, wearing clothing that is tight around the waist, which causes the blood supply in the lower part of the body to pool in the legs; standing in one place for long periods; prolonged sitting and habitually crossing one's legs, and straining from constipation. Women with varicose veins often have feelings of fatigue, heaviness, aching, burning, throbbing, cramping, and restlessness of the legs.

Like most women who try to hide their prominent leg veins, Ann-Marie wore compression stockings, bought panty hose in shades darker than her skin, and used camouflage makeup on her legs. But the process of applying makeup was messy, "so I just settled for wearing pants, even to fancy occasions," she said. Until, that is, she heard about the lunchtime option of getting rid of her leg veins forever.

questions and answers about leg vein treatments

WHAT ARE SPIDER AND VARICOSE VEINS?
Spider veins are unattractive purple or red superficial leg veins that resemble a spider's legs, hence their name. The very tiniest are known as capillary telangiectasias. They are less than 0.2 millimeter in diameter, thinner than uncooked cappellini, and red or pink. They are the most responsive to laser therapy. The second type is called venous telangiectasias. They range from 0.2 millimeter to 2 millimeters in diameter (similar to a strand of uncooked spaghetti), and they are usually blue or red-blue. They

are most responsive to either sclerotherapy or laser treatment. *Varicose* veins are large, elevated, bulging blue or blue-green, and tortuous. They are responsive to sclerotherapy, surgery, or a new laser procedure called Endolaser.

WHO IS A CANDIDATE FOR LASER TREATMENT OF SPIDER VEINS?

Anyone who has true spider veins—*not* varicose veins. But people with Fitzpatrick skin types IV, V, and VI, or those with a recent tan, are not optimal candidates because they are at risk for excessive damage to their skin that may lead to crusting, blistering, hyperpigmentation, and scarring. This is because the laser's beam of light is distracted by the melanin in the skin and so fails to reach the deeper pigment in the blood vessels.

WHAT LASERS OR LIGHT SOURCES ARE USED TO TREAT SPIDER VEINS?

Most of the lasers and light sources that are used to treat broken blood vessels on the face can also be used for leg veins (see Chapter 14, "Laser Treatment of Red Problems"). Newer lasers with longer pulse durations and longer wavelengths, which are commonly used for laser hair removal, are also effective in treating leg veins (see Chapter 13, "Laser Treatment of Unwanted Hair"). Popular laser and light sources include Sclerolaser, Vbeam, VersaPulse, CoolGlide, Medlite, Photoderm, Vasculight, and Multilight.

HOW DO I PREPARE FOR MY PROCEDURE?

Think ahead! Don't wait until summer—when you'll dread wearing shorts and a bathing suit—to have your leg veins treated. It may take three to five sessions to treat each problem area, and the bruising or discoloration after you're treated will take time to fade. Avoid the sun; the treatment cannot be performed safely on suntanned legs. On the day of treatment, don't apply moisturizer, a sunblock, or makeup to your legs. Remove the hair on your legs ahead of time to give the doctor an unobstructed view of your veins. You might even consider having your leg hair removed by laser (see Chapter 13, "Laser Treatment of Unwanted Hair").

HOW IS THE PROCEDURE PERFORMED?

The leg veins targeted for treatment are identified and the skin is prepped with an antibacterial cleanser. You will be given goggles to protect your eyes from the laser's beam. Depending on which system is used, the skin is cooled either by a gel or a cooling device built into the handpiece of the laser. When the beam of light is delivered, it's attracted to hemoglobin, the red pigment in the blood. The light is converted to heat, which seals off the vessel and collapses the blood vessel wall. Eventually, the body reabsorbs the nonfunctioning vessel. The sensation from laser treatment may feel like a snapping rubber band, a splash of hot oil, or a needle being dragged along your skin.

WILL I NEED AN ANESTHETIC?

Usually not. EMLA cream can be applied to numb the skin, but for the most part the cooling gel, the chill tip on some machines, or a cooling spray (cryogen) is sufficient. Any discomfort is short-lived.

HOW WILL I LOOK IMMEDIATELY AFTER?

There may be some redness or bruising in the treated area and possibly a little swelling. Many doctors apply antibiotic ointment or steroid cream to the area. Occasionally some blistering or crusting of the skin occurs.

HOW WILL I FEEL IMMEDIATELY AFTER?
Like you made good use of your lunch hour!

HOW LONG DOES THE PROCEDURE TAKE?
If just a few small spider veins are treated, the procedure will take only a few minutes. If numerous veins are treated on the back of the knees, the thighs, and the calves, a session may take thirty minutes or longer.

HOW MANY TREATMENTS WILL I REQUIRE?
For maximum improvement, three to five sessions are usually necessary for each area. If one area is being treated, the interval between treatments is about four to six weeks since it takes that long for complete healing to take place. However, you can be treated more often if treatment is rotated to different areas; for instance, one week for the veins on your right leg, the next week for those on your left leg.

CAN LASER TREATMENTS BE COMBINED WITH OTHER PROCEDURES ON THE SAME DAY?
Laser or light therapy can be combined with sclerotherapy during the same treatment session. This often results in more rapid improvement and can reduce the total number of treatment sessions required. However, when both modalities are performed at the same time, there is an increased risk of skin breakdown and ulcer formation.

WHAT DOES THE RECOVERY ENTAIL?
You can return to normal activity immediately but avoid strenuous activity until the bruising goes away, which may take several weeks. Bruising may be helped by vitamin K cream and hidden

by camouflage makeup and opaque panty hose. Protect your legs
with clothing or sunscreen to avoid hyperpigmentation. If you
develop any darkening of the skin, a bleaching cream can help
to fade it.

HOW LONG WILL THE RESULTS LAST?

They may last for years. However, genes, obesity, and estrogen
are three powerful contributors to the condition, so it's always a
possibility that your spider veins will return. You may choose to
have maintenance sessions, but even if you don't, your legs will
look better after your treatment than they did before.

WHAT DOES THE PROCEDURE COST?

A single treatment may start at several hundred dollars; a series
may cost several thousand. Doctors usually base this fee on the
length of time the treatment takes, the number of laser pulses
delivered, or the surface area being treated.

WHAT ALTERNATIVE METHODS CAN BE USED TO TREAT SPIDER AND VARICOSE VEINS?

Compression stockings. Although these stockings don't eliminate leg veins, they improve circulation and reduce discomfort.
They may also help prevent additional spider veins from forming. In recent years manufacturers have responded to the fashion
desires of baby boomers, who wouldn't be caught dead in the
thick ugly stockings their grandmothers wore, by improving
the appearance of support hose. Support hose are also helpful
for pregnant women. During early pregnancy, blood volume
increases and hormones stretch out the blood vessels to hold the
blood. Women with a history of varicose veins should start wearing support hose as soon as they learn they are pregnant.

   Sclerotherapy is among the leading cosmetic procedures in the United States, with more than 500,000 treatments performed annually. A tiny needle is used to inject the veins with a chemical that irritates the lining of the vein, causing it to collapse. Eventually the body reabsorbs the nonfunctioning vessel and it simply disappears. A typical treatment involves several injections and lasts about twenty minutes. After sclerotherapy, however, tiny clusters of magenta-colored blood vessels called telangiectatic matting may appear as a side effect of treatment. Lasers and other light sources can treat this fine matting. Some of the chemicals used in the treatment may cause momentary stinging, burning, or leg cramps. If a small amount of the solution accidentally seeps outside the vessel into the tissues, an ulcer may form. Occasionally, temporary hyperpigmentation may occur. After the procedure, the legs are usually wrapped for a few days with a compression dressing to maintain the constriction of the vessels. Normal activity can be resumed immediately after the procedure.

Ambulatory phlebectomy (*phleb* = "vein," *ectomy* = "removal") is an outpatient surgical procedure using local anesthesia. A series of tiny nicks are made in the skin along the path of the damaged vein, from which the superficial varicose vein is pulled out. After the vein has been removed, a bandage or compression stocking is worn for a short period. If the veins are quite large, a Doppler ultrasound examination determines which blood vessels have incompetently functioning valves. If the examination reveals that the problem lies at the junction between the superficial and deep vein systems, vein stripping of the entire vessel may be indicated.

Vein stripping is usually performed by vascular surgeons while the patient is under general anesthesia. A special instrument, a stripper, is used to tunnel under the skin and remove the saphenous vein along its longitudinal axis. The ends of the damaged vein are tied off, and the vein is extracted like a long strand of spaghetti. When a person has throbbing, cramping, dull aching, stinging, burning, or leg pain in conjunction with certain

Doppler findings, vein stripping is sometimes the only treatment that produces relief. Significant discomfort follows the procedure and recovery can take up to two weeks. Definitely not for your lunch break!

Radiofrequency occlusion (closure) procedure, approved by the FDA in 1999, is an alternative to vein stripping and much less invasive and painful. A narrow catheter is inserted through a small incision behind the knee. With the aid of ultrasound, the catheter is threaded through the saphenous vein to the spot where the blood vessel links up with the deep venous system near the groin area. As the catheter is pulled back, the radiofrequency device that sits at the end of the catheter delivers energy to the vein wall, causing it to heat, collapse, and seal shut. This outpatient procedure is done under local anesthesia and takes about forty-five minutes. After it is completed, a bandage or compression stocking is placed on the treated leg. Normal activities can be resumed immediately, but patients must wear support hose for a week. There may be tenderness along the vein and bruising for a week or more. Complications include minor nerve damage, skin burns, and blood clots.

Endolaser is a brand-new technique, performed with local anesthesia. It is similar to the radiofrequency occlusion procedure but uses a laser instead of a radiofrequency device. A fine fiber-optic laser is inserted through the catheter and used to seal off the saphenous vein from the inside out. The Endolaser has not been cleared by the FDA to treat varicose veins, although it has been approved for other purposes.

In times past, women suffered with unsightly leg veins because treating them was so painful and expensive. Today, laser technology has made leg vein removal more effective, safer, quicker, and the perfect solution for women on the run!

part four

instant beauty and beyond

not-so-instant beauty

*some "instant" procedures—chin
and cheek implants, breast
enlargement, eyelid lifts, and
liposuction—require a longer
recovery period, but can still
be performed on your
lunch break*

Are you thinking about having your eyelids lifted, your breasts enlarged, your breasts reduced (if you're a man with gynecomastia), your chin or cheeks implanted with contour-enhancing materials, or the appearance of your skin dramatically improved with a deep chemical peel? If you're like most people, the only thing holding you back is the thought that many of these procedures are lengthy and complicated. Or perhaps you believe that they require a commitment of time you simply don't have. Or you're afraid of hospitals.

Well, you can throw away those concerns! While these procedures may not result in instant beauty, they can still be performed in a doctor's office on your lunch break—but they do require a recovery period of about a week or more.

Regina had become somewhat of an expert in improving "the whole package." At fifty-five, after raising three children, working as an assistant professor of mathematics in a southern university, and taking care of her aging parents before they died, she explained that she "was so used to meeting everyone else's needs that I just about forgot about myself."

When a friend detected that Regina was depressed, she recommended her to a psychotherapist. "I knew she meant well," Regina said, "but I instinctively knew that it was my body and not my mind that needed fixing." With her academic training, she embarked on a methodical search to find out what it would take to "fix" the things that were bothering her.

"For one thing, I hated the way my eyelids drooped and made me look sleepy and old," she said. "I thought my skin belonged on someone ten years older than I am. And most important, I truly couldn't stand my saggy little breasts. When I was younger, I used to envy women with bouncy, sexy breasts and plenty of cleavage, but I'd say to myself, 'Someday, those breasts will sag!' Ha! Now it's me who's sagging. I don't care if I'm in my fifties—I'm determined to get the breasts I've always wanted!"

Regina's search yielded plenty of information, the most surprising of which was that the procedures she wanted took so little time to perform. "I decided to devote a whole summer, from June to September, to reinvent myself," she said. "But by mid-July, I was already the new me!"

blepharoplasty

WHAT IS BLEPHAROPLASTY?

It's the medical term for an eyelid lift, surgery on the *upper* eyelids to remove excess (or redundant) skin, bulging pockets of fat, wrinkling, and a small amount of muscle in the area where women typically apply eye shadow. Often, the excess skin causes a hooded look, hanging down to such a degree that it rests on the eyelashes and causes people to appear downright exhausted.

Blepharoplasty can also be performed on the *lower* eyelids, either with an incision immediately under the lower eyelashes or from the inside of the lower eyelid (transconjunctival blepharoplasty). The former removes excess skin, wrinkling on the lower eyelids, and bulging pockets of fat. The latter is appropriate in younger people who have only a small amount of cosmetically unattractive fat to be removed but no excess skin.

HOW DO PEOPLE DEVELOP POCKETS OF FAT IN THEIR EYELIDS?

The eyeball sits in the bony orbit of the skull like a ball in a socket, surrounded by muscles, tendons, and ligaments that support and protect it but weaken as we age. The eyeball is also cushioned by fat that, over time, begins to bulge forward into the eyelids. In the upper eyelid, this is most prominent in and above the eye's inner corner and in the lid itself. In the lower eyelid, the "bags" under our eyes are, in fact, the bulging fat as well as an excess of wrinkled skin. While the aging process accounts for changes in the appearance of our eyelids, heredity also plays a major role, hence the bags under the eyes that are sometimes seen in people in their twenties and thirties.

WHO IS A CANDIDATE FOR BLEPHAROPLASTY?

For upper eyelid surgery, any person who has droopy overhanging lids that compromise the appearance, interfere with vision, or obscure the area where eye shadow is applied is a good candidate. Lower eyelid surgery is a helpful procedure for anyone who wants to get rid of wrinkled excess skin, puffiness, and bags.

ARE THERE HEALTH CONSIDERATIONS THAT WOULD DISQUALIFY ME OR INCREASE MY RISKS FOR THIS PROCEDURE?

These procedures may not be recommended for people with uncontrolled high blood pressure, thyroid disease, blepharitis (acute inflammation of the eyelids), dry-eye syndrome, or a history of ophthalmologic problems such as retinal disease. If you have preexisting eye or eyelid problems, you should have an eye checkup with an ophthalmologist prior to surgery.

HOW DO I PREPARE FOR BLEPHAROPLASTY?

To minimize the risk of bleeding, discontinue alcohol consumption and avoid vitamin E, aspirin, and aspirin-containing products as well as nonsteroidal anti-inflammatory drugs like Motrin, Advil, or Aleve for two weeks prior to (and also after) the procedure. Also stop or curtail smoking because it affects wound healing by constricting the blood vessels. On a less clinical note, it's a good idea to buy a nice pair of sunglasses to conceal any bruising and protect against the sun after surgery.

HOW IS A LOWER EYELID LIFT PERFORMED?

The ultrapulsed CO_2 laser is the ideal tool for transconjunctival lower blepharoplasty. The procedure is usually reserved for people in their thirties and forties who have a small amount of bulging fat under their eyes but not a lot of excess skin. After an intravenous sedative is administered, the cornea is numbed with a couple of drops of anesthetic and the eyeball protected by a dull metal shield. Then an incision is made through the conjunctival lining on the inner aspect of the lower eyelid and the laser simultaneously seals off any bleeding. The excess fat is exposed, teased out, and removed.

In people with an excess of wrinkled skin and bags under the eyes, an incision is made under the lower eyelashes and the fat is repositioned rather than removed. This is because as we age, fat in the lower eyelids diminishes, and removing it runs the risk of leaving the patient with a gaunt or skeletal look. The muscles of the lower eyelid are also repositioned and then tightened. The outer corner of the eyelid is elevated, excess skin is removed, and the area of incision is closed with stitches that either dissolve on their own or are removed in a few days following surgery.

HOW IS AN UPPER EYELID LIFT PERFORMED?
Preparation for an upper eyelid lift is the same as for lower eyelid surgery. In this procedure, an incision is made in the natural crease of the upper eyelid so that any scar is nicely hidden when the eye is opened. Excess skin, muscle, and bulging fat are removed from the upper eyelids, and the incision is closed. As in the lower eyelids, the sutures either dissolve or are removed a few days following surgery.

WHAT WILL I LOOK LIKE IMMEDIATELY AFTER?
You will have some swelling and bruising in the area around the eye, and you may feel a little groggy from the IV sedation.

WHAT DOES THE RECOVERY ENTAIL?
You will have to apply ice-cold compresses on and off for forty-eight to seventy-two hours. In a week or less, your doctor will remove the stitches. Swelling and bruising that can be covered by makeup may continue for several days but will diminish significantly by the second week. You will be able to return to your normal domestic and career life in five to ten days, and you can prepare light meals and do other nonstrenuous things during that

time. Strenuous physical activity, including sex, should be post-poned for at least two weeks. However, you can be out and about—wearing your new sunglasses!—within days after the surgery. Occasionally, there may be temporary tearing or dry eye symptoms that last for several weeks, but they can be helped with artificial tears.

ARE THERE ALTERNATIVES TO THE PROCEDURE?

Sometimes, a drooping brow can make the eyelids appear as if they too have excess skin—even when they don't. In this case, when the brow is surgically lifted, the eyelids are revealed to be in fine shape. In other cases, both the brow and the eyelids droop and surgery is performed to lift both. However, a brow lift is a lengthier procedure, definitely not for your lunch break!

HOW LONG DOES THE PROCEDURE TAKE?

Both upper and lower eyelid surgery can be performed in an hour.

CAN THIS PROCEDURE BE COMBINED WITH OTHER PROCEDURES?

Blepharoplasty is often combined with a brow lift or facelift, which are more complicated procedures that take longer than an hour to complete.

HOW LONG WILL THE RESULTS LAST?

Although the aging process doesn't stop, the benefits of blepharoplasty surgery often last from seven to ten years.

WHAT DOES THE PROCEDURE COST?
For blepharoplasty on the upper and lower eyelids of both eyes, the cost is generally in the $5,000 to $6,000 range, plus additional costs for the use of the facility and anesthesia.

facial implants

Facial implants are typically sought by parents who desire more balance or harmony in the shapes of their teenage children's faces, often because of underdeveloped chins or cheekbones that the children are born with. In older people, the chin or cheekbones may have undergone demineralization that changed the shape of their faces, or they may simply want to correct an imbalance they had lived with all their lives. Whatever the motive for facial implants, they restore the face to a more youthful and symmetrical shape.

CHEEK IMPLANTS (MALAR AUGMENTATION)
This refers to the enhancement of the malar (or cheek) bones. In this procedure, the cheeks are made fuller as the cheekbones themselves are augmented or enhanced. After local anesthesia and IV sedation are administered, an incision is made inside the mouth (where the upper lip joins the upper gums) and the implants, which are made of a soft, rubbery silicone material, are inserted under the facial muscles directly onto the cheekbones. The incision in the mouth is closed with stitches that dissolve. To avoid food getting caught in the incision and the risk of infection, minor dietary restrictions must be observed for about a week after surgery. If cheek implants are inserted as part of other cosmetic facial procedures like a facelift, brow lift, or lower eyelid surgery, they can be placed through an incision used for these procedures.

CHIN IMPLANTS

If a weak or recessive chin is associated with other lower jaw or dental occlusion problems, a chin implant alone will not solve the cosmetic problem and it might require more complicated jaw surgery. If the problems are solely cosmetic, however, a chin implant can provide enhancing shape to the chin. In the procedure, local anesthesia and IV sedation are administered, and the implant is placed through the same kind of incision in the mouth that is made for cheek implants—in this case, where the lower lip joins the lower gums. When a facelift is being performed at the same time, the incision under the chin, used to help rejuvenate the neck, may also be used to place the chin implant; stitches are removed in five to seven days. The implant is placed directly on the chinbone, under the muscles, and in a tight pocket. This helps to accommodate the implant's size and shape as well as to prevent migration. After the incision is closed, postsurgical dietary restrictions must be followed for several days. Both cheek and chin implants can be performed in an hour in an outpatient setting. While there may be minimal bruising and swelling following the procedures, patients can return to work almost immediately. The results are long lasting to permanent. Sometimes, an implant that is placed in a teenager or young adult is removed and replaced with a new implant during later adulthood. Both chin and cheek augmentations, when not performed in conjunction with other facial surgery, cost in the range of $3,000 to $4,000 each, plus anesthesia and facility fees.

chemical peels

Superficial peels using fruit acids give the skin a blushing glow but they don't get rid of significant wrinkles (see Chapter 8, "Feeling Refreshed with Chemical Peels"). Medium and deep peels, on the other hand, penetrate the skin more deeply, thereby producing long-lasting skin changes, including the production of new collagen and elastin.

TRICHLOROACETIC ACID (TCA) PEELS

These use 25, 30, or 35 percent acid concentration and are performed with the patient receiving IV sedation, general anesthesia, or no anesthesia at all—depending on whether concurrent procedures are being performed and what percentage of TCA is being used. If performed without any anesthesia, the person usually experiences a mild to moderate stinging sensation as the acid is applied to the skin. TCA peels are effective in treating medium-depth wrinkles and pigment variations in the skin that result from aging and sun damage. But they can cause scarring if they reach too deeply into the skin and be ineffective if they don't reach deeply enough. Recovery generally takes a week to ten days, and after that the skin will be a pink color, which usually lasts for about one to two months but can be covered with camouflage makeup. The cost ranges from $2,000 to $3,000. As with all cosmetic procedures, the skill and experience of the practitioner are paramount.

PHENOL PEELS

Performed under IV sedation or general anesthesia, these penetrate the skin more deeply and reliably than TCA peels. They must be applied slowly because when phenol seeps into the skin, it may induce an irregular heartbeat or, very rarely, cause kidney problems. This is why patients are hooked up to a cardiac monitor and have their vital signs checked closely throughout the procedure. Phenol can also cause permanent hypopigmentation in which the skin appears extremely white. Again, after the initial two weeks of downtime, the skin will be pink for two or three months, but camouflage makeup can be worn. The cost ranges from $5,000 to $6,000.

dermabrasion

Instead of acid, dermabrasion uses a handheld, rapidly rotating wheel studded with tiny diamond particles or a wire brush to sand the top layers of the skin and to reach deeper wrinkles and acne scars. Before the procedure, patients are often prescribed antibiotics and antiviral medications and advised to apply Retin-A, AHAs, or other agents that promote healing. The healing process may involve oozing and crusting of the skin, but within two weeks most people are able to apply makeup and resume their normal schedules.

Like deep chemical peels, dermabrasion poses a significant risk of permanent hypopigmentation and scarring, particularly in areas of the skin that are thin. In addition, because dermabrasion is a bloody procedure, it places the physician at increased risk for blood-borne infections, including hepatitis and HIV, and also obscures the operative field, making it difficult to control the depth to which the rotary device penetrates and therefore to determine its effectiveness in treating deep facial wrinkles. For all these reasons, many doctors prefer laser resurfacing to deep chemical peels or dermabrasion.

laser resurfacing (or peeling)

In this popular method of skin rejuvenation, a beam of laser light vaporizes the top layers of skin. The heating of the tissue stimulates a blanket of new collagen to form in the dermis that smoothes the skin dramatically and eradicates deep wrinkles and scars. The procedure, which can be performed in an hour, is more accurate and precise and the results more predictable than those achieved with dermabrasion or a chemical peel.

The carbon dioxide (CO_2) laser yields results that are similar to a deep phenol peel but without the cardiac and kidney risks and with more physician control of the procedure. Resurfacing facial skin with this high-energy pulsed or scanned laser was FDA-approved in 1994, immediately gaining widespread popularity among dermatologists and plastic surgeons, many of whom prefer the laser over TCA and phenol peels and dermabrasion. The good news is that the laser effectively erases moderate and deep facial wrinkles and improves the appearance of depressed acne scars. In fact, it often takes ten to twenty years off one's appearance. The bad news is that the treatment requires a good two weeks of recovery and the skin remains pink for two to three months. Patients love the results of CO_2 laser resurfacing but the prolonged downtime associated with the procedure makes it no free lunch!

Erbium:YAG laser resurfacing is somewhat analogous to the medium-depth TCA peel. While the improvement in deep wrinkles is not as dramatic as with the CO_2 laser, recovery and therefore downtime are significantly shorter. A singular benefit of this laser is that darker-skinned people have a lower risk of developing postoperative hyperpigmentation. The new generation of long-pulsed erbium lasers can achieve results equivalent to that of the CO_2 laser but with less downtime. The cost for full-face CO_2 or erbium:YAG laser resurfacing ranges from $5,000 to $7,500, including anesthesia and facility costs.

If you desire facial resurfacing but can't afford the downtime, it's wise to consider a series of lunchtime treatments with a *nonablative* laser (see Chapter 12, "Nonablative Lasers for Wrinkles").

coblation

Coblation (or electrosurgical cold ablation) is a new technology for skin resurfacing using electromagnetic energy as opposed to laser light. Known commercially as Visage, coblation is effective in treating *mild* to *moderate* wrinkles and sun damage in people with all skin types including those with dark skin. Treatment results in collagen contraction and skin tightening similar to that achieved by the erbium laser, but with a slightly shorter recovery period of from five to seven days. The mild redness fades within one month.

breast enlargement

Women who seek breast augmentation want to enhance their body's contour, correct a reduction in breast volume after pregnancy, or achieve breast symmetry. Ideal candidates are healthy, have no personal or family history of breast cancer or autoimmune diseases, and are nonsmokers.

ARE BREAST IMPLANTS SAFE?

While a raging controversy existed for many years about the possibility that leaking silicone accounted for autoimmune diseases in some women, studies over the past several years have not substantiated these claims. Currently, silicone gel–filled implants are available only to women participating in approved scientific studies. Implants are usually filled with saline (a salt-water solution) and have a silicone outer shell. They have been used for more than twenty-five years, closely monitored by the FDA. There is no scientific evidence about any relationship between breast implants and cancer.

ARE THERE ALTERNATIVES TO BREAST IMPLANTS?

Exercise can enlarge the pectoralis major muscle, which can give a woman the appearance of a slightly more prominent bust-line. Creams that are advertised to increase the size of the bust-line do nothing but decrease the size of your wallet. Padded and push-up bras, known generically as wonder bras and miracle bras, can provide the illusion of generous endowment. And *Sex and the City* faux nipples, known as nipple perks, can be, well, titillating.

A new device, called the Brava Breast Enhancement and Shaping System, an external suction cup device worn on the breasts for ten to twelve hours a day for ten weeks, has been reported to yield modest increases of less than one cup size. A more controversial method is fat injections into the breasts, a procedure that is largely frowned upon by most members of the medical profession. When fat is transferred from one part of the body to another, it often calcifies (hardens) in its new location and can easily be misinterpreted on a mammogram as breast cancer and a biopsy may be necessary. Clearly, the anxiety, nervousness, and apprehension associated with this nightmare scenario should be avoided.

HOW IS THE IMPLANT PROCEDURE PERFORMED?

The procedure, which takes less than an hour, is performed under general anesthesia or with IV sedation and local anesthesia. The surgeon makes a short incision in the breast crease (where the breast meets the chest wall), around the areola (the dark skin surrounding the nipple), or under the arm. Then the skin and breast tissue are lifted to create a pocket—either directly behind the breast tissue or, most often, underneath the chest wall muscle—for each implant. The implant is positioned in the proper site and then inflated with saline until the desired size is obtained. The incision is then closed with sutures and a dressing applied.

HOW WILL I LOOK IMMEDIATELY AFTER MY BREAST AUGMENTATION?

The breast area will be larger and swollen and there will be some bruising and soreness. Bruising lasts up to two weeks and the swelling gradually diminishes over the first month.

WHAT DOES THE RECOVERY ENTAIL?

For the first two to four days, recovery involves rest and pain control. Most normal activities, including a return to work, can be undertaken after four to six days, but strenuous athletics or anything requiring exertive arm motions should not be done for about four weeks. Within several days, the gauze dressings, if you have them, will be removed and your surgeon may recommend that you wear a surgical bra. Many surgeons also advise postoperative massage of the newly placed implants. If the implant shell is smooth, as opposed to textured, massage is usually initiated several days following surgery. This ultimately yields a softer, more natural-appearing breast and may also lessen the risk of capsular contracture—a squeezing or tightening of the capsule surrounding the implant that causes the implant to feel hard. You may also experience a burning sensation in your nipples for about two weeks, but this will subside as bruising fades. The stitches will come out in one to three weeks, but the swelling in your breasts may take two to four weeks to disappear, so your breasts may temporarily appear larger than you anticipated.

ARE THERE SCARS FROM THE SURGERY? WHERE ARE THEY LOCATED?

Small scars from the incisions are usually located under the breasts. They will be firm and pink for about six weeks but begin to fade over a period of months. Eventually, there will be a thin, nearly inconspicuous line. Also, you may experience some numbness near your incisions that usually, but not always, disappears over time.

WILL THE IMPLANTS AFFECT MY SEX LIFE?

For about two to three weeks, your breasts may be oversensitive to touch or stimulation. When the postoperative soreness diminishes after three to four weeks, you will respond as you did before surgery, although many women report that they feel sexier with their enlarged breasts and enjoy an enhanced sex life. However, in some instances, the nipples may become more or less sensitive than they were before surgery.

HOW LONG WILL THE RESULTS LAST?

Breast augmentation is permanent unless the implant ruptures or a decision is made to remove the implants.

WHAT ARE THE LIMITATIONS, RISKS, OR COMPLICATIONS?

Occasionally, a capsular contracture may occur if the capsule around the implant begins to tighten. This may cause the breast to feel hard and require the removal (and subsequent replacement) of the implant. In addition, breast implants may break or leak. When a saline-filled implant breaks, it deflates over a period of a few hours and the body absorbs the fluid.

WILL THE SURGERY AFFECT BREAST EXAMINATIONS?

For routine mammograms after breast augmentation surgery, it is important that you go to a radiology center that offers the kind of special techniques required to get reliable X rays and additional views of breasts with implants. Ultrasound examinations are often recommended for women with implants in order to detect breast lumps and to evaluate the implant. Regular examinations by your plastic surgeon and gynecologist are also important because women who have breast cancer detected early have enhanced prospects for survival. A woman can perform breast self-examination after augmentation, but she should wait for about a month until the swelling and tenderness have subsided.

WILL THE SURGERY AFFECT MY ABILITY TO GET PREGNANT OR TO BREAST-FEED?

There is no evidence that breast implants affect the ability to get pregnant or to breast-feed.

WHAT QUESTIONS DO I NEED TO ASK WHEN SEEKING A DOCTOR TO PERFORM THIS PROCEDURE?

- What experience have you had in performing breast augmentation?
- Can I see examples of your work in photographs taken of other patients?
- Are you willing to put me in touch with another patient who has had the procedure?

WHAT DOES THE SURGERY COST?

The cost ranges from approximately $4,000 to $8,000, depending on geographical location. Health insurance companies don't consider the procedure medically necessary and therefore don't cover its costs.

WHAT IS THE SATISFACTION RATE?
Breast augmentation is the third most commonly performed cosmetic surgical procedure in the United States, after liposuction and blepharoplasty. Overwhelmingly, women who have breast augmentation are thrilled with the result.

breast reduction in men

Gynecomastia, enlargement of the male breasts, is a condition that is either idiopathic (cause unknown) or associated with certain medications, excessive alcohol intake, and diminished liver function, the use of anabolic steroids, or excessive use of marijuana. The condition is common, although usually temporary in adolescent boys when male breast tissue is developing. If the condition persists during adolescence or occurs as an adult, then breast reduction is indicated. Breast reduction involves removing overdeveloped glandular breast tissue or fatty tissue or both. Overdeveloped glandular tissue is removed through a small incision in the areola (around the nipple). Fatty tissue is removed with liposuction through a small incision under the arm or at the edge of the areola. The procedure usually takes an hour under local anesthesia with IV sedation or general anesthesia. Then an Ace bandage or elasticized garment is wrapped around the area. There is tolerable discomfort after the procedure, and swelling and bruising last for a week or maybe two, during which strenuous upper-body exercises should not be performed. Stitches are removed in one to three weeks. Generally, gynecomastia surgery costs about $4,000, plus anesthesia and facility fees.

liposuction

WHAT IS LIPOSUCTION?

This most popular cosmetic surgical procedure in the United States helps sculpt the body by removing unwanted fat from the hips, abdomen, buttocks, thighs, knees, upper arms, chin, cheeks, and neck. While diet and exercise can often bring about a great shape, liposuction is effective in removing areas of fat that stubbornly resist every weight-loss method.

WHO IS A CANDIDATE?

People of normal weight who have firm skin but pockets of fat that just won't go away in spite of their best efforts. While older people can benefit from the technique, their skin has less elasticity and so the results may not be as satisfactory.

ARE THERE HEALTH CONSIDERATIONS THAT WOULD DISQUALIFY ME OR INCREASE MY RISKS FOR THIS PROCEDURE?

The procedure is not recommended for those who have diabetes, heart or lung disease, or poor circulation, or who have recently had surgery near the area to be contoured. Interestingly, a recent study showed an improvement in insulin levels in insulin-resistant diabetics who underwent large-volume liposuction (greater than five liters of fat removed).

HOW IS LIPOSUCTION PERFORMED?

A tiny incision is made in the area to be suctioned and a narrow tube or cannula is inserted that vacuums out the fat layer beneath the skin. The cannula is repeatedly pushed and pulled back and forth to break up the fat cells and suction them out.

Since fluid is lost along with the fat, you will receive intravenous replacement fluids.

ARE THERE ALTERNATIVES TO CONVENTIONAL LIPOSUCTION?

Newer and refined methods of the technique include:

Tumescent technique involves injecting a medicated solution of saline, lidocaine, and epinephrine (that constricts blood vessels) into fatty areas before the fat is removed. The solution facilitates fat removal, reduces blood loss, provides anesthesia both during and after surgery, and reduces postoperative bruising.

Super-wet liposuction is similar to the tumescent technique but it uses less fluid.

Ultrasound-assisted lipoplasty (UAL) uses ultra-high-frequency sound wave energy that passes through the fat areas causing the walls of the fat cells to rupture and then liquefy, after which the fat is removed with liposuction. UAL is particularly effective in fibrous areas of the body like the upper abdomen, back, saddlebags, or the enlarged male breast. When the ultrasound energy is applied *internally*, sound waves are emitted from the tip of the cannula as it passes through the fat, resulting in "melting" of the fat that is then sucked out by liposuction. When the ultrasound energy is applied *externally*, the medicated solution is administered to the area to be treated and a probe (similar to the one used in sonogram tests during pregnancy or for the diagnosis of gallstones or kidney stones) is rubbed over the skin in the same area, after which the melted fat is removed with small cannulas, only in lesser quantities than when internal ultrasound is used. Recovery from the external ultrasound procedure is more rapid than recovery from the internal ultrasound procedure.

WHAT ARE THE LIMITATIONS, RISKS, OR COMPLICATIONS?

While liposuction is considered very safe when performed by an *experienced* plastic surgeon, there are risks that include:

- Infection and delayed healing
- The formation of fat clots or blood clots that may migrate to the lungs and cause death
- Excessive fluid loss that can lead to shock
- Friction burns or other damage to the skin or nerves
- Perforation of the vital organs
- Adverse drug reactions

To diminish the likelihood of complications, it is important to check the credentials of your plastic surgeon and to be sure that the facility in which you have the surgery is accredited. (See Chapter 4, "Better Safe Than Sorry.")

WILL I NEED ANESTHESIA?

Liposuction that removes only a small amount of fat on a limited number of body sites can be performed on a lunch break with local anesthesia numbing only the affected areas. This is often combined with IV sedation to keep you calm. More extensive liposuction requires more time and usually general or regional anesthesia.

WILL I HAVE SCARS?

Usually scars from liposuction are small and placed strategically so they're hidden from view.

WHAT WILL I FEEL LIKE IMMEDIATELY AFTER LIPOSUCTION?

You may feel stiff and sore and experience some pain that can be alleviated by pain medication. You may also have burning, swelling, bleeding, and temporary numbness or pigment changes. In addition, you may experience some fluid drainage from the incisions. A special elastic garment is worn for several weeks following surgery to enhance skin contraction and redraping of the skin over your new shape. Your doctor may also prescribe antibiotics to prevent infection.

WHAT IS THE HEALING PROCESS LIKE?

The stitches from the incisions either dissolve or are removed by the doctor in about seven to ten days. You should start to walk around as soon as possible to reduce swelling and to help prevent blood clots from forming in your legs. But avoid strenuous activity for two to four weeks. Most of the bruising and swelling usually disappears within two to three weeks, but some swelling may remain for six months or more. It is often helpful to have a series of Endermologie treatments (see Chapter 10, "Banishing Cellulite") following liposuction because they help to diminish postoperative swelling and allow you to enjoy your new shape that much faster.

WHAT IS THE SATISFACTION RATE?

If you have realistic expectations and do not anticipate that you will look like a Victoria's Secret model, you will be very happy with the results. You will see a noticeable difference in the shape of your body quite soon after surgery. You won't have the protruding fat deposits that bulge out from your slacks or skirts and you'll feel much more comfortable in your own skin.

afterword

So there you have it. Now you know what your youthful-looking friends—the ones who promised to age gracefully—are really doing. They're all engaging in the new form of "cheating": having "quickies" during lunch—quick-fix cosmetic procedures, that is. Isn't it time for you to indulge yourself, too?

We hope we have given you all the vital information you need to feel confident about the choices you make. Go ahead, "do" lunch! Allow yourself to get gorgeous and enjoy your new self-esteem and instant beauty.

glossary

ablation Removal of thin layers of tissue.

Accutane Brand name of isotretinoin, a derivative of vitamin A, a medication used to treat cystic acne.

acne Inflammatory disease of the oil glands of the skin, especially of the face or back.

actinic keratosis Precancerous scaly, rough, red patch that may progress to squamous cell carcinoma.

aesthetician Person trained in methods to enhance beauty.

age spot Flat, brown discoloration on the skin that results from overexposure to the sun and aging; also called sunspot or liver spot.

allergy Hypersensitivity or reaction to environmental factors or substances such as foods, dust, or medication.

alopecia Loss of hair.

alpha hydroxy acids (AHAs) A family of chemical exfoliants that are nontoxic antiaging "fruit acids" derived from fruits, sugarcane (glycolic acid), and sour milk (lactic acid).

ambulatory phlebectomy Outpatient procedure in which superficial varicose veins are removed through tiny nicks in the skin along the path of the vein.

anesthesia Total or partial loss of sensation induced by an anesthetic.

angiofibroma A tiny pink bump on the face made up of blood vessels and collagen.

angioma Tumor or lesion composed of blood vessels.

antiandrogen Topical over-the-counter agent such as Ethocyn that promotes smoother, more supple skin.

antibacterial Any agent that is effective against bacteria.

antibiotic A drug that is effective against bacteria.

antioxidant A chemical compound that reduces oxidation, thus combating the aging process, damage to DNA and RNA, autoimmune diseases, cancer, and other maladies.

autoimmune Production of antibodies against one's own cells or tissues.

azelaic acid A topical medication, also known as Azelex, commonly used to treat acne and to lighten dark spots on the skin.

basal cell Cell found at the base, or bottom, of the epidermis.

basal cell carcinoma The most common form of skin cancer. Caused by the uncontrolled growth of basal cells of the epidermis damaged by exposure to ultraviolet light.

beauty mark A mole or nevus.

Becker's nevus A flat, light-brown, cosmetically disfiguring discoloration that usually develops during puberty and adolescence, typically on the torso and upper extremities.

benign Noncancerous.

beta hydroxy acids (BHAs) A family of chemical exfoliants that have antiaging effects with minimal irritation.

birthmark A mole or blemish that is present on the face or body at birth.

bleaching agent Medication that slows or blocks the production of melanin in the skin to lighten age spots, fade blotchiness, and help erase dark circles under the eyes.

blemish Any mark or discoloration on the skin that mars the appearance.

blepharitis Acute inflammation of the eyelids.

blepharoplasty A procedure in which a crescent of skin, muscle, and some underlying fat are excised from the upper or lower eyelid to correct drooping or sagging; also called an eyelift.

body dysmorphic disorder A psychiatric condition in which those afflicted become preoccupied with an imagined defect in their appearance.

Botox A substance derived from the bacterium *Clostridium botulinum* that is injected into underlying muscles in the forehead and around the eyes to reduce muscle-related wrinkles.

bronzer A self-applied cosmetic that gives the skin a tanned appearance.

brow lift A surgical procedure to elevate the brow and permanently smooth forehead wrinkles; also called a forehead lift.

café-au-lait spot A benign flat, light-brown to tannish lesion that may be associated with neurofibromatosis.

camouflage makeup A flesh-toned product used to cover scars, bruises, and discolorations of the skin; also called masking foundation.

capillary A minute blood vessel that connects an artery to a vein.

cellulite The rippling, cottage-cheese-like appearance of subcutaneous fat that protrudes from the thighs, buttocks, and hips.

chemical peel The application of an acid to the skin to smooth wrinkles and even out blotchiness.

cherry angioma A benign bright-red vascular bump commonly occurring on the trunk of adults.

chilling tip A device attached to the handpiece of a laser that continuously cools the treatment site and diminishes pain.

cleanser An agent that removes oily residue, makeup, dirt, and dead skin cells.

collagen The main structural protein in the dermis.

complexion The natural color, texture, and appearance of the skin.

concealer A cosmetic used to cover blemishes and neutralize pigment irregularities; also called primer or neutralizer.

congenital nevus Pigmented lesion in the dermis that is present at birth.

cosmeceutical A hybrid that combines features of both a cosmetic and a pharmaceutical.

crow's feet Radiating lines around the eye that result from aging and normal facial expressions such as squinting.

cryosurgery Freezing with liquid nitrogen to destroy unwanted tissue.

depilatory An agent capable of removing hair.

dermabrasion Treatment for smoothing the surface and textural abnormalities of the skin, including severe acne scarring, that involves the use of a high-speed rotary device and sander.

dermatology Medical study and treatment of the skin, hair, and nails.

dermis The layer of the skin beneath the epidermis comprised of a tough matrix of collagen and elastin that anchors and supports the lymph vessels of the immune system as well as blood vessels, sebaceous glands, sweat glands, nerves, and hair follicles.

diode laser A small portable laser that is efficient and cost effective.

dynamic cooling device An apparatus that emits a short burst of cooling agent milliseconds before each pulse of the laser, thereby reducing pain and thermal damage.

dynamic wrinkles Creases in the skin caused by movement and facial expressions that contract the underlying muscles.

dysplastic nevus An atypical mole that may be a precursor of malignant melanoma.

elastin Connective tissue found in the dermis that contributes to the skin's resilience and elasticity.

electrolysis The process of eliminating excess hair by inserting a needle into each hair follicle to destroy the hair bulb with a weak current of electricity.

electromyography A technique used by doctors to locate the correct muscle into which to inject Botox.

EMLA cream A topical anesthetic.

emollient An agent that smoothes, softens, and moisturizes the skin.

endoscope A surgical device for seeing the inside of the body through a tube with an attached camera and light source.

epidermal nevus A benign brownish, pebbly textured birthmark usually located on one side of the face, arms, or legs.

epidermis The outer, protective layer of skin.

estrogen Female sex hormone produced by the ovaries, adrenal glands, placenta, and fat.

excimer A laser used to treat various skin conditions.

excise Remove by cutting, either with a scalpel or laser.

exfoliant An agent that causes the outer layer of skin cells to slough off.

extrinsic aging Changes in the skin due to sun exposure; also called photoaging.

eyelift See **blepharoplasty.**

facelift A surgical procedure to rejuvenate the appearance of the face and neck in which underlying muscle structures are repositioned, fatty deposits are removed, and skin is pulled up, redraped, and tightened.

filling agent A substance such as collagen, silicone, or one's own fat that is injected into the skin to fill in wrinkles, acne scars, and other skin depressions.

finasteride FDA-approved oral drug, also known as Propecia, for the treatment of baldness.

Fitzpatrick skin types An evaluative system developed by Dr. Thomas Fitzpatrick to assess skin color and a person's tendency to tan or burn.

folliculitis Inflammation of the hair follicle.

forehead lift See **brow lift.**

foundation makeup A liquid cosmetic containing pigment tones that covers the skin with a sheer, even look and gives the skin a matte (flat) finish or pearlized shimmer.

free radicals Free-floating electrons resulting from oxidation that have been linked to the aging process, damage to DNA and RNA, autoimmune diseases, cancer, and other maladies.

glabellar lines Vertical forehead creases between the eyebrows.

glycolic acid A "fruit acid" derived from sugarcane with exfoliating properties; used for superficial chemical peeling.

graft A piece of skin (or other tissue) excised from one place on the face or body and transferred to another.

gynecomastia Enlargement of male breasts.

hair follicle A deep, narrow canal with its enclosed developing hair.

hemangioma A proliferative vascular lesion that originates from blood vessels during embryological development and is found in approximately 10 percent of infants.

hemoglobin The oxygen-bearing component of red blood cells that gives the blood its red color.

hormone A chemical substance produced by glands that is conveyed through the bloodstream and affects other tissues.

horny layer The topmost layer of the epidermis; also called the stratum corneum.

hydrocystoma A benign tiny, clear, fluid-filled growth on the face.

hydroquinone A bleaching agent that slows or blocks the production of melanin to lighten age spots, fade blotchiness, and help erase dark circles under the eyes.

hyperhidrosis Profuse sweating.

hyperpigmentation Darkening of the skin through overproduction of melanin.

hypertrophic scar A scar that is thickened, raised, or elevated.

hypoallergenic Designed to reduce the chance of allergic reactions.

hypopigmentation Lightening of the skin.

ice-pick scar Deep scar left over from acne or chicken pox.

immune system A complex system involving certain fluids and organs of the body that is responsible for fighting infection and defending the body against foreign invaders.

implant A synthetic material that is placed in the body to augment the shape of breasts, cheeks, and chin, among other body parts.

inflammation Redness, swelling, and pain as a result of irritation, injury, or infection.

intravenous sedative Tranquilizing or calming medication that is given directly into the vein through intravenous tubing.

intrinsic aging Changes in the skin such as loss of elasticity due to the chronological passage of time.

isotretinoin The active pharmacological ingredient in Accutane, a vitamin A derivative prescribed for cystic acne.

jowl Accumulation of fat and sagging excess skin along the jawline.

keloid A raised, fibrous scar that extends beyond the original margins of a wound.

Kenalog A steroid medication that decreases inflammation.

keratin A protein substance that forms the outer layer of skin, nails, and hair.

keratinocyte A cell in the epidermis that produces keratin; also called a squamous cell.

kojic acid A bleaching agent that lightens dark spots on the skin.

laser An acronym for *l*ight *a*mplification by *s*timulated *e*mission of *r*adiation.

laserbrasion A precise method of vaporizing layers of the skin with the laser to create a smooth surface and improve the appearance of acne scars and wrinkles; also known as a laser peel and laser skin resurfacing.

laser-generated airborne contaminant Substance that has been shown to have mutagenic and carcinogenic effects and can cause ocular and upper respiratory tract irritation.

laser peel *See* **laserbrasion.**

laser sculpting Using a laser to remove thin layers of tissue to reshape and recontour a body part such as the nose.

laser skin resurfacing *See* **laserbrasion.**

lesion A pathological change in the tissues, such as a skin growth or an inflammatory condition.

lidocaine A local anesthetic that is given by injection into the skin.

lipoplasty *See* **liposuction.**

liposuction A technique of body contouring or body sculpting in which unwanted fat is removed from areas such as the abdomen, hips, and thighs by the use of a suction (vacuum) device and small tubes (cannulas) inserted via tiny incisions.

lipstick bleed lines Deep, vertical lines that radiate around the area of the mouth as one ages; particularly common in those who smoke.

liquid nitrogen Dry ice that when applied to the face acts like an exfoliator.

liver spot *See* **age spot.**

lupus A connective tissue disorder that mainly affects young women, causing flushing of the cheeks and nose among other signs and symptoms.

marionette lines Creases that extend from the corners of the mouth to the jawline.

mask Skin agent with a base of clay, mud, cream, or oil that removes sebum from oily skin, helps unclog pores, hydrates dry skin, and provides some degree of exfoliation.

masking foundation *See* **camouflage makeup.**

melanin The skin or hair pigment that accounts for variations in skin or hair color.

melanocyte A cell in the skin that contains melanin.

melanoma A malignant and potentially deadly form of skin cancer.

melanosome The tiny body within the melanocyte that contains melanin.

melasma A patchy brown skin discoloration, usually on the face, also known as chloasma or the "mask of pregnancy."

metronidazole A topical drug, also known as MetroGel or Metro-Cream, that kills mites and is used to treat rosacea.

micropigmentation The art of tattooing tiny amounts of colored pigments into the skin; also called permanent makeup.

minoxidil A topical over-the-counter drug, also known as Rogaine, used to retain or restore hair.

moisturizer An agent that softens and smoothes the skin by locking in natural water content.

mole A benign growth on the skin that is usually pigmented; also called a nevus.

nasolabial folds Smile or laugh lines that extend from the nostrils to the corners of the mouth.

nevus *See* **mole.**

nevus of Ito A bluish-gray, benign skin blemish on the shoulder or upper arm that is found in the dermis; more common in those of Asian descent.

nevus of Ota A bluish-gray, benign skin blemish on the face and in or around the eye; more common in females of Asian descent.

nevus spilus A light-brown lesion with a sprinkling of confettilike dark-brown pigment speckles found on the trunk and extremities.

nonablative laser A resurfacing laser that eliminates wrinkles without any peeling of the skin.

nonacnegenic Not stimulating the formation of whiteheads or pimples.

noncomedogenic Not causing blackheads.

papillary dermis The upper portion of the dermis.

pH The measure of the acidity or alkalinity in the solutions of certain skin products.

pharmaceutical An FDA-approved drug that, in the case of the skin, has been proved to alter its structure and function.

phenol An agent used to achieve a deep-level chemical peel to treat wrinkles and acne scarring.

phlebectomy *See* **ambulatory phlebectomy.**

phlebitis Inflammation of the veins of the legs.

photoaging *See* **extrinsic aging.**

plantar wart A viral growth commonly occurring on the bottom of the foot.

plastic surgery Molding or reshaping various features for aesthetic and reconstructive purposes.

poikiloderma of Civatte A condition characterized by a flushed, blotchy, red neck.

pores Tiny openings in the skin that serve as exit routes for sweat and oils, regulate body temperature, and from which hairs emerge.

port-wine stain A congenital overabundance of tiny blood vessels beneath the surface of the skin. Of unknown etiology, the malformation may vary from light pink to deep purple.

postoperative Period of recovery and healing that takes place after a surgical procedure has been performed.

pseudofolliculitis barbae Ingrown hairs on the face and neck and most common in men of color.

psoriasis A chronic, noncontagious skin disease characterized by inflammation and pink, scaly patches.

pulse duration Length of time during which a flash of laser light is emitted.

pulsed light A beam of light emitted in a short burst of energy with minibreaks in between.

radiation The emission of light waves or particles.

red-nose syndrome An acquired condition characterized by a gradually enlarging, reddened, and misshapen nose with enlarged pores, the result of skin and sebaceous gland overgrowth and a proliferation of blood vessels; also called rhinophyma.

Renova FDA-approved prescription skin cream containing the vitamin A derivative tretinoin that has proved to reduce fine wrinkles, surface roughness, and brown spots associated with sun exposure and aging.

reticular dermis The deep level of the dermis where the deepest wrinkles and ice-pick acne scars reside.

Retin-A A topical medication derived from vitamin A, also known as tretinoin, that is used to treat acne and photoaging. It is the same product as Renova, but not in an emollient base.

rhinophyma *See* **red-nose syndrome.**

rhinoplasty Surgical modification of the nose; also called a nose job.

rosacea A condition causing flushing, dilated blood vessels, and pustules on the nose and cheeks.

scalpel A surgical knife.

scar A permanent mark that remains on the skin after an injury or wound.

scleroderma A connective tissue disorder causing hardening of the skin among other signs and symptoms.

sclerotherapy Injection of an irritating chemical into the vein that causes the vessel to collapse and ultimately disappear.

sculpting Reshaping tissue.

sebaceous gland Oil gland in the skin.

sebaceous hyperplasia Benign bumps on the face made up of an overgrowth of oil glands.

seborrheic keratosis Light-tan to dark-brown wartlike growth that appears to be "stuck on" the surface of the skin, a condition most common in older people.

sebum Oil from sebaceous glands.

self-tanning agent A cosmetic that artificially stains the skin.

silicone A filling agent that is no longer used due to problems with migration and foreign body reactions.

silicone gel A dressing placed over a raised scar to soften and flatten it.

skin graft *See* **graft.**

skin tag A benign fleshy growth commonly found on the neck, under the arms, and in the groin.

spider angioma A cluster of tiny blood vessels that emanates from a central point.

spider vein A tiny purple or red superficial leg vein, so named because it causes streaks in the skin that appear to be as fine as a spider's legs.

squamous cell See **keratinocyte.**

squamous cell carcinoma A form of skin cancer caused by the uncontrolled growth of squamous cells of the epidermis that have been damaged by exposure to ultraviolet light.

steroid Anti-inflammatory drug.

stratum corneum See **horny layer.**

stria Stretch mark.

subcision A technique in which fibrous bands that anchor a depressed scar are severed to release the tethered scar tissue.

sunblock A thick, opaque cream that physically reflects the sun's rays away from the body.

sun protection factor (SPF) A number used to indicate the effectiveness of sunscreen in preventing redness or sunburn.

sunscreen A skin-protective agent that chemically absorbs the sun's harmful ultraviolet radiation.

sunspot See **age spot.**

sweat gland A gland that secretes perspiration through a pore in the skin.

syringoma A tiny benign bump derived from sweat glands around the eyes and on other areas of the face.

tattoo A permanently etched or ingrained mark or design in the skin made from various colored pigments.

telangiectasia A tiny, superficial "broken" blood vessel.

tissue splatter Tiny fragments of tissue containing viable cells and organisms that may disseminate into the air during a laser procedure.

toner A cosmetic agent that removes excess oil and temporarily "tightens" the skin; also called clarifying lotion, refresher, astringent, or purifier.

topical Pertaining to a medication that is applied externally to a particular part of the body.

transconjunctival blepharoplasty A procedure to remove excess fat from the lower eyelid that does not involve an outside skin incision.

trauma A wound or injury.

tretinoin The active ingredient in Retin-A and Renova.

trichloroacetic acid (TCA) An agent used to achieve an intermediate-level chemical peel to treat wrinkles, sun damage, acne scarring, and pigmentation problems.

trichoepithelioma A benign bump around the nose.

turkey neck Excess skin and fat under the chin.

ultraviolet light A portion of the electromagnetic spectrum associated with high-energy, short-wavelength light that is invisible but has the ability to damage chromosomes and cause skin cancers.

vaporize To convert into barely visible mist or vapor.

varicose vein Abnormally dilated leg vein.

vascular Pertaining to vessels such as veins, arteries, and capillaries that circulate blood throughout the body.

vein stripping The surgical removal of varicose veins.

venous lake A benign small blue nodule often found on the lower lip that is filled with deoxygenated (venous) blood.

vitiligo An autoimmune disorder in which the body attacks the pigment cells and leaves the skin mottled with stark white spots.

wart A benign bump on the skin caused by infection with the human papilloma virus.

wrinkle A furrow, ridge, line, or crease on the skin.

xanthelasma Yellowish fat deposits in the skin around the eyes, sometimes associated with elevated levels of cholesterol.

resources

Accreditation Association for Ambulatory Health Care, Inc.
3201 Old Glenview Road, Suite 300
Wilmette, IL 60091-2992
847-853-6060
Fax: 847-853-9028
E-mail: info@aaahc.org
Web: www.aaahc.org

American Academy of Dermatology
1350 I Street, NW, Suite 880
Washington, DC 20005-4355
202-842-3555
Fax: 202-842-4355
Web: http://www.aad.org

American Academy of Facial Plastic and Reconstructive Surgery
310 South Henry Street
Alexandria, VA 22314
800-332-FACE or 703-299-9291
Fax: 703-299-8898
E-mail: aafprs@aol.com
Web: www.aafprs.org

American Academy of Micropigmentation
2709 Medical Office Place
Goldsboro, NC 27534
800-441-2515
Fax: 919-735-3701
E-mail: zwerling@micropigmentation.org
Web: www.micropigmentation.org

American Association for Accreditation of Ambulatory Surgery
    Facilities, Inc.
1202 Allanson Road
Mundelein, IL 60060
847-949-6058
Fax: 847-566-4580
E-mail: aaaasf@sprynet.com
Web: www.aaaasf.org

American Board of Medical Specialties
1007 Church Street, Suite 404
Evanston, IL 60201-5913
866-275-2267
Fax: 847-328-3596
Web: www.abms.org

American Medical Association
Data Services Department
515 North State Street
Chicago, IL 60601
800-665-2882
Fax: 312-464-4184
Web: www.ama-assn.org (look for Physician Select)
This site will tell you about a doctor's license, training, board certification, etc. For $60, the AMA will send you profiles of five doctors.

American National Standards Institute
1819 L Street, NW, 6th Floor
Washington, DC 20036
202-293-8020
Fax: 202-293-9287
E-mail: ansionline@ansi.org
Web: www.ansi.org
The ANSI document Z136.3, titled "National Standards for the Safe Use of Lasers in Healthcare Facilities," has become the accepted national benchmark for laser safety and is the guideline used by OSHA, JCAHO, and most professional organizations' standards for practice.

American Society for Aesthetic Plastic Surgery, Inc.
11081 Winners Circle, Suite 200
Los Alamitos, CA 90720
888-ASAPS-11
Web: www.surgery.org

American Society for Dermatologic Surgery
930 North Meacham Road
Schaumburg, IL 60173-6016
847-330-9830
Fax: 847-330-1135
Web: www.aboutskinsurgery.com
Consumer hotline: 800-441-2737

American Society for Laser Medicine and Surgery
2404 Stewart Square
Wausau, WI 54401
715-845-9283
Fax: 715-848-2493
E-mail: information@aslms.org
Web: www.aslms.org

American Society of Plastic Surgeons
444 East Algonquin Road, Suite 110
Arlington Heights, IL 60005
847-228-9900
Fax: 847-228-9131
Web: www.plasticsurgery.org
ASPS Plastic Surgery Information Service: 888-475-2784

Food and Drug Administration
Center for Devices and Radiological Health
1350 Piccard Drive
Rockville, MD 20850
301-443-4690
Fax: 301-443-8818
E-mail: dsma@cdrh.fda.gov
Web: www.fda.gov
This agency establishes mandatory standards for the manufacture of lasers.

Food and Drug Administration
Center for Food Safety and Applied Nutrition
Office of Colors and Cosmetics
200 C Street, SW
Washington, DC 20204
202-401-9725
Contact if you experience a reaction you believe is related to a cosmetic product.

International Society of Hair Restoration Surgery
930 North Meacham Road
Schaumburg, IL 60173-6016
847-330-9830
Fax: 847-330-0050
E-mail: cachziger@aad.org

Joint Commission on Accreditation of Healthcare Organizations
1 Renaissance Boulevard
Oakbrook, IL 60181
630-792-5000
Fax: 630-792-5005
Web: www.jcaho.org

Laser Institute of America
13501 Ingenuity Drive, Suite 128
Orlando, FL 32826
800-34-LASER or 407-380-1553
Fax: 407-380-5588
E-mail: lia@laserinstitute.org
Web: www.laserinstitute.org

Lupus Foundation of America, Inc.
1300 Piccard Drive, Suite 200
Rockville, MD 20850-4303
800-558-0121 or 301-670-9292
Fax: 301-670-9486
E-mail: info@lupus.org
Web: www.lupus.org/lupus

National Alopecia Areata Foundation
710 C Street, Suite 11
San Rafael, CA 94901
415-456-4644
Fax: 415-456-4274

National Psoriasis Foundation
6600 SW 92nd Avenue, Suite 300
Portland, OR 97223-7195
800-723-9166 or 503-244-7404
Fax: 503-245-0626
E-mail: getinfo@npfusa.org
Web: www.psoriasis.org

National Rosacea Society
800 South Northwest Highway, Suite 200
Barrington, IL 60010-9802
888-NO-BLUSH
Fax: 847-382-5567
E-mail: rosacea@aol.com
Web: www.rosacea.org

National Vitiligo Foundation, Inc.
611 South Fleishel Avenue
Tyler, TX 75701
903-531-0074
Fax: 903-525-1234
E-mail: vitiligo@trimofran.org
Web: http://www.nvfi.org

Occupational Safety and Health Administration (OSHA)
Directorate of Safety Standards
U.S. Department of Labor
200 Constitution Avenue, NW
Washington, DC 20210
202-219-8061
Fax: 202-219-6064
Web: www.osha.gov

Skin Cancer Foundation
245 Fifth Avenue, Suite 1403
New York, NY 10016
800-SKIN-490 or 212-725-5176
Fax: 212-725-5751
E-mail: info@skincancer.org
Web: www.skincancer.org

index